I0449143

No Matter What

Based on a true story

Latonya R. Baskerville

Copyright © 2014 by Latonya R. Baskerville
First Edition – February 2014

ISBN
978-1-4602-2807-4 (Hardcover)
978-1-4602-2808-1 (Paperback)
978-1-4602-2809-8 (eBook)

All rights reserved.

Copyright 2012, All rights reserved

No part of this book may be reproduced, stored in a retrieval system, or transmitted by any means without the written permission of the author.

No part of this publication may be reproduced in any form, or by any means, electronic or mechanical, including photocopying, recording, or any information browsing, storage, or retrieval system, without permission in writing from the publisher.

Produced by:

FriesenPress

Suite 300 – 852 Fort Street
Victoria, BC, Canada V8W 1H8

www.friesenpress.com

Distributed to the trade by The Ingram Book Company

Table of Contents

Latonya R. Baskerville Dedication

To my parents Leroy and Patricia Baskerville: I love you both so much. You showed me that a couple in love could accomplish many things through hell and high water. And through your inspiration, I am still praying and waiting for the kind of man who will be able to recognize that I am that virtuous woman as described in the Word of God.[1] Mommy and Daddy, you have made me extremely proud and grateful to be your firstborn. I know I am not exactly what you wanted me to be, but our Father made me better.

To my children Tyshawn, Janera, Joquan: I thank you all for your patience, support, and encouragement during the crazy, chaotic times in my life. I am so grateful for you. I took y'all through for more than a decade of your lives, and I promise to be the best mother I can be and to continue to support and encourage y'all though your trials, errors, and accomplishments. In Jesus' name, amen. To my other daughter Shaquisha Yodatt Foulks, I love you very much Thank You for allowing me in your life, I must admit its never a dull moment.

To my granddaughter Shanice Baskerville and her mother Nysha Onnie Fauntleroy: I am so grateful to God every day for having y'all in my life. It's not easy being on the other side of parents' disputes, but thank God you allowed me to be the voice of reason to keep our family together, no matter what.

To my honey dady Lawrence L. James: I can't believe how much we have endured in other relationships to wind up back together again. I have always loved you, but falling in love with you conquers all, hands down. You allowed me inside of you, and I am amazed every day with your talents, sensitivity, affection, support, encouragement, and love for me. I am extremely grateful to God for protecting our bond despite the rejection we experienced from others.

To my godchildren Jahnai and Cheahn: God placed y'all in my life in a special way, and I placed you in my heart, where you'll stay.

To my grandma Jeanelle Childs: I thank you for all the love, comfort, commitment, and support you gave to my mentally ill mom. I feel blessed and highly favored to have received your spiritual teachings and special love. You always prayed for and blessed others without casting judgment, treating them in your home when they were suffering from the effects of drugs, alcohol, and mental instability. Now, I am following in your footsteps by continuing to give that special love back to my community, and I have taught my children to do the same. I love you, Grandma.

To my other mother Jesstine Baskerville: I appreciate all your tough love and encouragement. When you first came into my dad's life, I thought you were trying to erase the memories we had of my mother. I was wrong; instead, you strengthened them. You are tough and loving, like my mom. And just like her, you speak your mind and tell the truth, no matter what. Thank you, Ma, for planting the seeds for my authorship. You gave me a book to read and purchased the tapes and recorder to get me started on my books. Thank you so much for believing in me before I believed in myself.

To my brother Leroy Jr. (RIP) and my son Shayquan (RIP): Thank you for all the memories and love you left me with. I know you're smiling down on me from up above with the rest of God's angels.

To my sisters Keyonda, Jazzette, Tiffany, Shanta, and Nicole: Y'all are the best sisters in the world! You have always loved and cared for me, no matter what my life challenges have been. I was able to fight every obstacle that Satan threw my way because I had all of you to talk to and laugh with. Thank you so much, babies!

To my nieces Imani, Fatimah, Tatyana, Atallah, Lakiya, Tamiya and to my nephew Kenneth (aka Butta), NaQuan, Timothy, Leslie to my cousins Shanecqua, Jeanelle, Kevin Poole (aka The Wave), Landa, Buttons, Boobie, Linda (RIP), Poppa, D. J., Brian, Kareem, Michael, Chantz, E. J., Anthony, Audrey, Boo, Freda, Maurice, Kevin, Tiffany, Eric, Delisa, Shakenna, Isaac, Nina, Calvin, Crystal, Claudette, Brenda, and David Jr.; to my aunts Jackie, Millie J. Poole, Ada, Hilda, Bert, Tracy, Lori, Sally, Debra, and Liz; to my uncles Jimmy (RIP), Aries, Michael, David, Kevin Sr., Kemp (RIP), and William (RIP): I thank you all for your love and support.

To my personal mental supports Denise, Lorna, Valerie (aka The Professor), Bertha, Cindy, Roxy (aka Buddy), Dr. Maia, Lareesha, Maria C., Marie, Jennie, Dennis, Sonia, John, Cy, Taneille, Lashauna, Kelly, Yolaine, Gloria, Panthea, Shamika, Budy, Alex, Melissa N., Loretta W., Todd, Maricol, Pat, Else, Ronica W., C. J., Marisa, Lola, and to all my A.N.G.E.L.S.: There were so many days when you listened to me without casting judgment or blame. Oh my God, what would I have done without you? I don't dare think about it.

To my keepsake children Jerry, Tanaisha, Cheryl, Ebony, Tasha, Naquan, Rasheed, Terence, Dannie, "Mszjuicybaby," Jay, Rayniece, Allen, and Diana: Y'all kept me up praying all the time for your parents and your safety. I spent time listening to you and making suggestions because I wanted to ensure that this world wouldn't conquer you. I love y'all something special.

To my Village Mothers; Thank you for your Love, Ms Doll, Ms Smith, Ms Hammond.

To my Village Mothers that are gone but never forgotten; Ms Queeny, Ms Florence, Ms Stella, Ms Pressely and Ms Terry.

Acknowledgments

To the NYC Administration for Children's Services, the Bronx Treatment Court, Cumberland Diagnostic and Treatment Center, and the HOPE Program: Thank you very much for your stern and structured service plans that built me into a fully productive and valued member of society and my community.

To the Jewish Child Care Association: Thank you for your support, encouragement, training, and overall love. Coming from a foster care agency, this was a very unusual practice. But it has paved the way for the level of treatment that can be received by clients who seek services at Training Individuals Make Better Attitudes, Inc., where I am the executive director.

To my mentors Candace T., Carmen G., Keturah P., Charles P., Richard A., Mike S., Margaretta Y., Anna M., Joseph J., Francis A., and Ruth C.: Thank you all so much. You've shown me real leadership and how to work side by side to help others become leaders on the frontlines. Your passion and support have compelled me to be the best leader I can be and to help others do the same.

To my friends and Not Alone Fellowship members Dupree, Nate J., R.I.P. to David W., Antoinette B., Charles C., Greg, James, Dawn K., Sophia, Linda, Debbie P., Lindra, Vanessa, Antwone J., Angel and Marianne Lady CoCo, Shabazz and

Alisha, Ben, Henry W., Dexter B., Supreme and Stephanie, Jeff, Monroe, Ruby and Terry, MaLora, Azzam, Octavius, George, Sam Bee, Hasheem, Robin C., Jerome (aka PeeWee), Rukaiyah L., Cynthia T., CeeCee, Fly Ty of 40 Block Photos, Pamela E., Joanne (aka Queeny), Ron da Bomb, Boo, June Bug, Miles Green, Nathaniel R., West, Real, Randy R., David R., Ty, Angel, Sha, Austin, Kareem T., Chink, Frank H., Darrell, John Steve W., John, Stan da Man, Gadior, Pattie and Ray of Pattie's Catering and LA Diva Productions, Pee wee Lisa, "Blessedbyhisgrace" Fanny, Capoo, Pop Latoya (aka Slim), Steven W., Diana, Paula, Country, Charm, Muzz Luv's pet service, Inger and Greg, Alverna S., Mia, Nana Gerri of GZ Productions, Bed-Stuy Ty, Jazi Jeni, Ella F., Kenny, Prince, Mr Gatior aka Samuel, Tonya and James, Adrienne F., Carlene and Shati, Michelle, Carita H., Al and Kelly, Mona, Dawn, Melissa R., Debbie C., Yvonne, Ina and Yusuf, Arianna W., Nadine, Doreen, Son Shyne, Naima R, Tifini L., Racquel C., Moe and Andrea Kirby, Kendell, Donna and Charles, Luz, Debbie T., Candy S., Pam D., Blacpearl Ruebin, Sugar, Reese, DeeDee, Terry W., Tamika, Monique P., Venus, Star, Ricky Barrino, Tisha, Mytish, Mr. Jackson (aka Watermelon Man), Yolanda S. (aka Cookie), Shamolly Rose, Dude, Bev, Nashaona W., Nasharah S., Malaki E., Mecedees, Shelly, Chimene, Saundra and Robert Taylor, Tina B., Wayne, Zack, and BooBoo: I placed your names on this very special list of people because you shared your stories and listened to mine. You encouraged my path and supported my journey, and I received a little piece of each and every one of you. I'm doing great things for God with my life now. I'm a productive member of my community, and I thank you all dearly for giving me such precious pieces of you. I love you all—please never forget that. If I have forgotten anyone, please forgive me. Even if I didn't mention you here, please know that I still need you in order to continue my God-given destiny.

To my community merchants and health care providers Gabby of Gabby Jewelry, Jay, Country from Halsey Street Barbers, Beverly's Beauty Blessings, Mr Jackson, the staff of Foodtown in Restoration Plaza in Bed-Stuy, Bed-Stuy Pharmacy, Kings County Hospital Center, Fulton Dental Plaza, Tony's Health Food Supermarket, Mike from Dynasty's Hair Salon, and Mr. Williams: I sincerely thank you all! Nigel Barbers, Joe's Cleaners and Bravo supermarket on Dekalb ave

To all my brothers and sisters on Halsey Street and Throop and Tompkins Avenues: Much love to you for all your comfort and workout encouragement.

To my TV pastors Bishop T. D. Jakes, Joel Osteen, Dr. Creflo Dollar, Joyce Meyer, and Joseph Prince. I give you all my special thanks. May God forever bless you all. Your daily teachings of the true Word of God have fed my spirit and nurtured my soul so that I can continue to carry out God's predestined will for my life.[2] Amen.

To my newfound church family of Mount Pisgah Baptist Church, pastored by Rev. Dr. Johnny Ray Youngblood: I am so grateful to be welcome in the house of the Lord again. I had felt like a fish out of water for so long. Mount Pisgah, you truly are one of the seven churches Christ is coming for. I love y'all so much.

To Total Recovery Church, Pastor Derrick E. Harvey, and Lady Fanta F. Harvey: I send you a very special thank you.

To my Public Assistance worker Ms Hart, Section 8 case manager Ms. Burnett and HASA case managers Ms.Oluyemisi Adeyemi and Ms .Audrey Duverglas: I send you all my special thanks. It might seem strange to show gratitude and apprecia- tion to you, but you truly deserve this and more. You helped me maintain a home for me and my son. You encouraged my goals, dreams, and entrepreneurship regardless of my health and financial situations. You kept my spirits high while I was going through a healing process. Sometimes, workers from these programs can be very nasty and negative. Thank God you were not. May God continue to bless you so that you can continue to be a blessing to others.

To New York's best landlords Slimey, The Telford family, Banana Kelly management, Mrs Adolphine, Yvette and Akil M.: Most authors probably wouldn't do this, but by now you should have figured out that I'm not most authors! I appreciate all of you for working with me through my extreme financial crises. I thank God for landlords like you, who really care about their tenants' well-being. May God bless you and those like you in everything you do.

To Kenny C., R.I.P to Debbie, Sable, and Charles from Rent-a-Center: I send you a special thanks for helping me keep proper, updated electronics in order to be able to write books even while under financial and medical distress. My writing has helped me feel the inspiration and empowerment of being able to encourage others. This has been so important to me.

To my Facebook family: OMG! You guys have helped me get through my surgeries and rehabilitation process. All your jokes, posts, and comments have made me feel so loved, supported, and respected. I love y'all so much and continue to look forward to your comments.

Foreword

by Janera Baskerville

I remember my mother having tea parties with me and my imaginary friend Carolla, whom I always told my mother I loved so much. This was when I was just four years old. My mother had bought me a beautiful pink-and-white tea set, complete with cups, a kettle, and teaspoons. We would spend hours together sipping tea and having playful conversations. We would even get dressed up in outfits that my mom made out of some of her old clothes. It seems only fitting, then, that now we have the opportunity to have another "tea party" here with other mothers and their daughters.

My mother, Latonya Baskerville, is a strong black woman with a beautiful heart. She has a terrific sense of humor, and often, the precious time we spend together is filled with laughter. In so many ways, my mom has been a great inspiration in my life because she has shown me that success is always an option if you put your mind to it. And by setting a shining example, she has proven to me that it is never too late to correct your mistakes. I thank God every day for blessing me with such a wonderful mother.

Mom was a drug addict for over ten years. As a result, my siblings and I were taken away from her by the Jewish Child Care Association. At the time, my older brother was ten years old, my younger brother was a newborn, and I was five. We were placed in my great-grandmother's home until my mother straightened herself out. Thankfully, we were there for only eighteen months.

Within a short time my mother was able to successfully complete her rehabilitation programs. She did so well that the agency offered her a full-time job as a parent advocate to help her get back on her feet. Since then, my mother has gone back to school and completed her CASAC-T credential in substance abuse. She is now on the board of directors for TIMBA Incorporated, a nonprofit organization that focuses on the needs of children, families, and at-risk youth in low-income communities.

My mother's success has influenced me in many ways. It has made me realize that I can overcome any obstacle, no matter how big or small it is. In fact, at the beginning of my first year at Acorn High School for Social Justice, I was not really motivated and had attendance and behavior issues. I used to cut school with my friends and get caught by school safety. I also used to sneak out of the house and go to parties until four in the morning.

But all the while, I could hear my mother's voice telling me, "Mooshie, you can correct any mistakes you make as long as you want to correct them for *you*." She even took time off from her professional career to help put me on the right track. And I did just that. My GPA at the beginning of the year was below 55 percent. Now, my GPA is above 80 percent. I no longer cut class nor do I go places I shouldn't go. I've learned that I have my whole life ahead of me. My focus is on being successful in school, being a good daughter, and being the best person I can be. All of this is thanks to the phenomenal role model I have in my mother.

Latonya Baskerville, mother of Janera Baskerville, deserves to be "Mother of the Year" because of her strength, humor, and inspiration. She wins my appreciation every day. My mother and I have a very open relationship—she's honest with me and I'm honest with her. That is why my love for her is so deep and valuable. I am so proud of my mother's success. I love her so much . . .

If only you knew.

Preface

To all my brothers and sisters, both young and old, of all races, creeds, religions, or lack thereof, I love you all very much. The story you are about to read is a token of my love for you.

Please be aware that this book includes explicit material as well as Bible scriptures (from the New International Version), which can be found at the end and are labeled throughout this book with numbers. I felt the need to be able to express the story of my life freely, honestly, and openly. I am not a pastor, preacher, deacon, prophet, or minister of any kind. I am just a regular, sinful human being who loves the Lord with all my heart and who truly appreciates all the grace, patience, and mercy He has shown me throughout my life. God is my savior and the only one who can judge me on everything I've been through and chosen to share here. So with all due respect, I ask that you keep an open mind while reading my book, and to please clean the beam out of your own eye before you clean the mote out of mine!

It was hard growing up in my community: for years, I was bullied, teased, and tormented about my weight, height, and dark-colored skin. At only thirteen years old I remember crying daily and asking God why my community hated me so much. Before I knew it, I had fallen into a dark hole, indulging in crime, sex, and drugs to gain acceptance from my bullies. But that didn't work—the bullying got worse, the drugs got weaker, and the cycle just got more complicated. I needed more money to get more drugs, so at seventeen, I started prostituting and allowing any man with money to do whatever he wanted to me, whether it was protected or unprotected. As the days went on, my "job" got harder and harder. I was raped, beaten, abandoned, and sexually violated. I even started smuggling drugs across the country and selling them around my community.

Then one day I made a direct sell to an undercover cop across the street from a public school. I was arrested and sent to jail. When I was brought before a court judge, he explained that the crimes I had committed were felonies and that I was facing two to six years in prison.

My legal aid attorney pleaded with the judge to grant me rehabilitation as an alternative to incarceration. This is when I started to turn my life around. I accepted and embraced rehabilitation. I was sentenced to a drug treatment program that I completed in August 1999, and then was referred to a job readiness program that I completed in June 2000. By this point, I was fully motivated to do good things for myself. I enrolled in a GED program, receiving my GED just a few months later, in October 2000. Soon after that I took up work for over ten years with the foster care agency that reunited me and my kids. Upon resigning, I founded a not-for-profit, wrote three books, composed seventeen poems, and just recently became a certified field producer for Brooklyn Public Network. I learned how to accept and deal with all the consequences of my destructive former lifestyle. And I made it my goal to continue renewing and healing myself by sharing my story with other girls so they don't have to follow the kind of destructive path I was once on. Girls like me, with stressful and painful beginnings, *can* have hope and happy endings.

The Word of God has been the blueprint for my happy and healthy lifestyle. I am forever grateful that He allowed me His knowledge and wisdom so that I could survive, learn from my mistakes, find my purpose, and become closer to Him. I don't expect to save everyone; Jesus Christ did that when He died on the cross. I simply follow God's Word to the best of my human ability and hope to encourage you to do the same.

This book is meant to help, guide, and offer support mostly to youths, and especially to young women who are coming of age and to pregnant teen moms. Of course, I welcome anyone and everyone to read my book, but I am particularly invested in young people. Having personally worked with troubled teens and their families for over ten years before I became disabled, I intend to continue working with them until my dying day.

Thank you very much for your time and for showing your support by reading my book. I pray that it helps you develop greater understanding as well as gain something productive that you can use in your life and the lives of your loved ones.

May God bless you.

Introduction

First and foremost, I would like to thank my Lord and Savior Jesus Christ for giving me two lives in one lifetime. This book describes all the heartaches, struggles, stressors, and pain that I went through before I became absolutely determined to live my life against all odds. Hopefully, after reading this, you will be inspired to have courage, determination, and endurance through your own trials, and you, too, will know what it means to have hope, faith, trust, and patience in God, no matter what!

The world today seems to deem any kind of behavior as acceptable in the eyes of God. Well, I beg to differ. But by no means am I judging anyone else's behavior.[3] I myself don't walk in perfection, so I cannot judge the behavior of others.[4]

Again and again, many so-called pastors, preachers, and prophets have misused and manipulated true believers of Christ. I apologize for these people's abuse of the Word of God. Those dishonest brothers and sisters are the very reason, though, that God told His children to study His Word.[5]

Many of us have been scorned and converted by these corrupt souls.[6] For hundreds of years, even though God was the one who helped our ancestors battle enslavement and discrimination, we turned away from Him, angry and upset. Instead of directing our resentment on our Lord and Savior, though, we should have recognized the false prophets and targeted our anger on them. Many of us have even seen our own family members misuse the Word of God. They have told us stories of the retribution God casts on us when we do not follow His ways. They have threatened us with stories of fire and brimstone punishments from God.

But I know, because He has showered me with his grace time and time again, that God's love is eternal and all-encompassing. His mercy, endurance, and patience are limitless. I thank God so much for having released His message to me to share with you. People might not always understand God—His ways are not human ways.[7] But what keeps us everlastingly connected to the Lord is our faith in Him.

God never leaves us. We leave Him when we become angry and afraid of being rejected by Him. We know when we've done wrong. So it is during those times that we should ask for forgiveness and try not to make the same mistakes again. I prayed to be saved from my drug and alcohol addiction—oh, I prayed for over sixteen years. Then one day, He delivered me. Trust me, I'm a *hot mess*, but I know that whenever I ask God to help me and to forgive my sins, He always comes through. The Lord loves all His children, and I dedicated my body, mind, and soul to Christ because I love Him.

Countless times He's blessed me, even when I probably didn't deserve it. For the longest time, just like so many others, I, too, trusted the words of false prophets. Even by reading the Kings James Bible, I still had no idea what God wanted from me. But eventually, despite the pain and shame I had to endure from those false prophets, I found the courage to go to God myself.[8] I asked Him to bestow me with the knowledge and understanding of His will for my life.[9] I struggled so much to get where I am now. But the Word of God was the blueprint I used to rebuild my life and gain back my good health.[10] I can't imagine what I would have done without it.[11]

I feared people showing hostility and banning me from my community for being so brutally honest about my experiences. But I knew God would bless me for obeying Him. In the end, my stressors became my victories: they gave me the opportunity to receive God's grace and mercy. And I know that if He did it for me, if you just believe in Him, He will do it for you, too.[12] My life is no longer just a life; it's a living testimony of the love, grace, mercy, and patience God shows all His children who believe in His only begotten Son, Jesus Christ.[13]

Never did I imagine that I would write a book about my life and weight loss success to help and guide others. I asked God, "Why do I have to tell the world *my* business?" The Lord reminded me that this was why He saved me. I argued, saying, "Father, who cares about all the miracles You showed me in my life?" But the truth is, people do care, because so many of them are dealing with these same kinds of situations in their lives right now. The obesity epidemic is solid evidence that people need help from God. I was obese for the majority of my life, and even I have never seen this many obese people before. If they had any idea of what kinds of problems excess weight causes, they would drop to their knees.

If you are reading this and are overweight or obese, remember that I've been there, too. Your weight issues are likely connected to more than just bad eating habits. You might even realize that you eat bad foods as a way of dealing with your hardships. It's a deadly and false perception that food can help heal you, especially when you're feeling sad, angry, or lost. May this book help you start to look at your life in a different way. May you be encouraged to go forward, no matter what your life struggles or stressors may be. I pray my book will help guide you in your personal life and give you the faith and courage to seek God in all that you go through.[14] He loves you and promised to do so always, no matter what.[15] May God bless you with love, grace, mercy, and peace. In Jesus' name, amen.

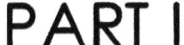

PART I

My Beginnings

I was born on October 18, 1969, to teenage newlyweds Leroy and Patricia Baskerville. My parents had been raised in the South during a time when it was widely believed that obese children were healthy children, so my love of food developed very early on. According to my dad, my mom never gave me baby food; I was fed grits and eggs instead, chewed straight from her mouth to mine, because in those days it was normal for many mothers to chew their babies' food before placing it into their babies' mouths. Until my brother Leroy Jr. was born two years later, I was the only child and my parents' sole focus. Once my baby brother was born, though, our family was complete.

I remember my mother and father being a great team. My mom was a nurse with a very demanding work schedule, so my dad would take me and my brother out every weekend. He felt it was important for our family to spend recreational time together even though my mom was always busy. We'd visit places like Coney Island, go roller-skating, and go on picnics. Dad would often also take me and Leroy Jr. to McDonald's, where we could enjoy eating whatever we wanted, no matter the size or cost.

But suddenly, my parents started having problems. They would argue for hours. My brother and I never knew what caused each argument, but whatever it was, it always resulted in my dad leaving the house. Things felt different whenever my dad was gone. So to cope, my brother and I would run rampant through the house, eating every sweet we could find. Whenever my dad returned, he would clean the house and notice his kids' reckless eating. This would lead to my parents having yet another argument, which would then lead to my dad leaving again.

My parents didn't like arguing in front of me and my brother, so they finally tried separating for a while to let things calm down between them. It was during this time that my dad went to Virginia. He was only in his twenties, and even though he had his mom and sisters there, he didn't have a married male role model to advise him on the commitment and patience it takes to maintain a marriage. So my dad ran blindly and created even more issues for himself. By the time he returned to my mom, other women had started writing him letters. When my mom found them, she began having a mental breakdown, accusing my dad of sleeping with every woman he met.

My father became increasingly frustrated, because he didn't know how to save his marriage. So he decided that a divorce would be better than arguing in front of me and my brother every day. We couldn't figure out what had happened to my mom. Why had she become so different? But whatever it was, my dad couldn't endure it at that young age. Soon, everything changed. Because my mom couldn't manage paying the mortgage by herself, the bank took our huge house. All the family furniture was placed in my grandmother's backyard shed, and over the years, the weather turned it into garbage. The pink canopy and oakwood bedroom sets . . . the hundreds of toys, books, clothes . . . all of it rotted away. Pretty soon, my grandmother Jeanelle took over the responsibility of caring for all of us.

My grandmother was a Baptist minister with a Southern upbringing. She had moved with her children to New York when they were young. The New York streets in the sixties were probably a scary place for my grandma. She had no street-life survival skills; her way of dealing with everything was through prayer and meditation. So she turned all concerns and issues over to my grandfather.

My grandfather, who was a military veteran and retired longshoreman, did know how to deal with street life. But he handled things with guns, so talking to him was useless. My grandma had learned very early on how to be a good home-maker and housewife because my granddad had been so caught up in the grips of New York's rough streets.

Even though my father was deeply saddened by the loss of his marriage, he always made it a point to stay in contact with his kids to make sure we were okay. I was a daddy's girl, and I remember memorizing my dad's work number so I could call him anytime. The sound of my dad's voice was enough for me to get by until I could see him on the weekends. My brother was a mama's boy, though, so he was still just fine with living around my mom.

I deeply admire and love both of my parents for all they did for each other and for their children. My dad would travel to see us through rain, sleet, and snow. He never disappointed us; when he said he would come at a certain time, he would always be there. Regardless of how he felt deep down, he tried his best to stay strong despite the breakup of his family. My dad managed to keep a smile on his face through it all, and because he smiled we smiled. During their marriage, my mom was also a wonderful provider and a great support to my dad. She accomplished so much by the age of only twenty-five and was the virtuous woman described in the Holy Bible.[16] So when my mom had her mental breakdown, my heart broke. I wish her family would have properly addressed her condition, but the fact is, in those days mental illness in African Americans was denied and ignored. Thank God for my dad, though. He never wandered off and abandoned his kids. He was always available for us.

By the time I was eleven years old and my brother was nine, we were both already incredibly obese for our age, and the community bullies reminded us of this daily. My parents' divorce and the loss of our home surely played a huge part in our eating habits. Food gave me a distorted feeling of comfort—eating a ham and extra cheese whole hero sandwich with gobs of mayo would make me feel better. Sugary snacks also soothed me. Unfortunately, unhealthy food was always readily available for us, too, and we got whatever we wanted. All we had to do was ask. Health-conscious living was not a part of our household, and fruits and veggies were never suggested as good snacks.

I weighed 276 pounds at the age of twelve and my brother weighed 175 pounds by the time he was ten. My grade school years are a bit foggy, and I don't really recall having much trouble during that stage. But I was the tallest and largest kid in the whole school, so the other children were probably afraid that I would beat them up or "sit on them" if they tried bullying me. That expression always bothered me, because I never did those kinds of things—I never *sat* on anybody. I didn't know how to fight and I didn't want to learn. All I wanted was to have real friends, be attractive enough to get a boyfriend, and go out to play. The background I was raised in did not teach me violence.

Soon my dad announced he would be remarrying. He wanted to get full custody of us and asked if we wanted to live with him and his new wife. I was happy to live with my dad; he had always been my link to life. My brother, on the other hand, wasn't comfortable leaving my mom, but he came along with us anyway. The custody hearing was simple, due to my mother's mental health condition, and after just two months in family court my dad got custody. So we went to my grandma's house, packed our clothes, and kissed my mom good-bye. Whereas I was extremely happy to be with my dad, my brother was not thrilled at all. He would miss my mom a lot.

The very day we got to my father's house, his new wife's son got very angry because he didn't want to share his room with my brother. This led to him jumping on my dad and the two of them fighting. I was enraged. Running to the kitchen, I grabbed a butcher knife and headed out to help my dad. His wife grabbed me and nearly got stabbed because I was so furious her son had laid his hands on my father. I remember crying and feeling very angry, because I knew right then that this was not going to be as wonderful as I had dreamed it would be. That day, my dad ordered his wife's son to leave his home and never return. And from that point on, my stepmother made our life a living hell, nitpicking about every single thing me and my brother did every single day. This was not a Cinderella story. No, this was real—we were now living with a wicked stepmother.

By the time I reached junior high, I weighed about three hundred pounds and was six feet tall. I was always so stressed out back then because I knew my dad's wife would be waiting at home to mentally torture me and my brother. This was a nightmare. I thought I would be happy living with my father, but instead I was miserable. Every day was like living in hell and walking on glass barefoot. Leroy Jr. and I didn't know how to be regular children in this home because if we made one wrong move, my dad would be notified. My father worked a tough job driving an eighteen-wheel tractor trailer, and I knew he didn't need any more stress while on the road. So to make things easier, I tried making friends in Queens to bide my time each day until my dad came home from work.

I managed to meet some fairly cool girls. But they weren't tall and extra large like me, and whenever boys came around, they would ditch me. I was built like the boys, and soon the girls were taunting me with names like "Audrey the Giant" and "Amazon." I couldn't understand why these girls hated and teased me; I never did anything to them. I wasn't attracting their boyfriends due to my physical appearance, so what was the problem? I never figured it out.

Once I realized that females had issues with me, I stayed far away from them. Boys became cool with me, though—I wasn't a threat to their brotherhood, and nobody was trying to fight for my hand or have sex with me. I loved being with the boys. They treated me with dignity and respect. I was allowed to listen to them talk about fly girls for hours. The things they would say helped teach me to be the best woman I could be for a man: I found out how to keep my womanhood fresh, nice, and tight, and I learned that if I trusted my man and gave him space, he would love me more than I could imagine. I discovered that all men are not dogs, and that if drugs are not involved, a man will not cheat on a woman he loves. I dreamed of having a respectable man of my own and being a mother to seven boys when I grew up.

Around this time, my father's wife finally wore him out with complaints about his children. In particular, she became frustrated and resentful that I didn't know how to be clean with my monthly. What she didn't understand or care about was that I had never learned about feminine hygiene because my mom was diagnosed with mental illness when I was just a child of eight. I was fourteen years old when my stepmother made us leave my dad's home. But I never held my dad responsible for the witch he had accidentally married to help him raise me and my brother. So we headed back to our grandmother and mom with our clothes in a garbage bag. By this point, all I knew was rejection. And I knew it well.

I remember my years in high school being a total nightmare. I was teased, bullied, and beaten up every day. I never understood why taunting and bullying other children was necessary; it wasn't like the ones who got bullied walked around tormenting attractive, popular children. I was called names like "Fat, Black, and Ugly," "Kamala" (the wrestler), "Black Giant," "Fat and Funky," "Amazon," "Gorilla," and "Sasquatch." It was as though every person in the whole school hated my appearance—even the teachers would take potshots at me. I dropped out after only two months because I couldn't handle the abuse anymore.

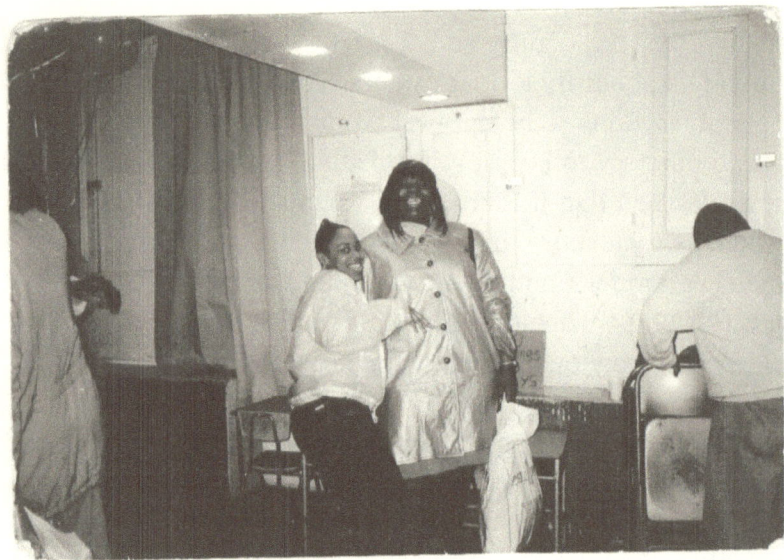

At fourteen, I started smoking weed. The popular children said it was cool, and in the beginning, it was. It also helped me cope with my feelings of rejection, loneliness, and low self-esteem. This was the beginning of my adolescence, and due to my mom's mental breakdown, there was no one to talk me through it. Sometimes I would assume I could talk to the other girls, but then the boys would come around and I'd realize I was wrong. As a result, my distrust for women became strong, because I saw time and again how they would flip the script. I had enough experience with female peers to know better than to hang with them too often. It was ironic: I always tried to encourage brothers to be loyal to their fellow sisters, but I never quite felt comfortable bonding with women because I knew that having male company would immediately make them change. Pointing out my body size, body shape, and skin color was always the first dagger they'd stick in my back. They never wanted the males to get attached or attracted to me. But they didn't seem to realize that teenage boys wanted trophies on their arms, not chicks who were considered ugly.

In the eighties, society didn't accept or respect people with obesity issues. If you were obese, you would become a bully, be bullied, commit suicide, or attempt to survive by hiding from others. I was often the hidden friend, because whoever was seen talking to me would get teased, too. Whenever I encountered bullies by themselves, they wouldn't say or do anything. It was only when they had an audience that they wouldn't shut up. That's when they would tell me I was not physically appropriate for boys my age; I was too big and too black, and nobody owned a zoo for a gorilla. Sometimes kids would even lie and accuse me of liking some boy. This was supposed to be a joke, but neither the boy nor I ever found it funny because he would then become angry and call me all kinds of mean names.

My grandmother wasn't able to guide me through this stage of my growth. She wouldn't discuss adolescent issues like fashion, peer pressure, sex, drugs, and pregnancy. They were out of her scope. So without any proper guidance, I started my journey down a very long, dark path. Money, I thought, would help me make friends out of my bullies, so I bought weed and alcohol, hoping that if I got them high, they wouldn't tease me. Well, that didn't work. They just laughed at and tormented me more because they'd be high and couldn't stop laughing even if they wanted to. Pretty soon, my grandma noticed I was spending a lot more money than she could provide, and I began having a really hard time getting money from her to buy drugs.

At fifteen, I met a boy who I believed loved me dearly. So I gave him my virginity, and he gave me my first pregnancy. This boyfriend was a great source for weed and munchies. But the problem was that he didn't have a job, so he got locked up regularly. By this time, I was so big for my age that I attracted old men. So whenever my boyfriend got locked up, I used this to my advantage for money. In the beginning, old men would buy me alcohol and weed, but when the money was low, I had to pretend I enjoyed alcohol only. Alcohol was not my favorite substance, but it helped me get through having to do sexual favors for these old men. By the time I was sixteen, neither weed nor alcohol was getting me high anymore. This was when I was introduced to crack cocaine.

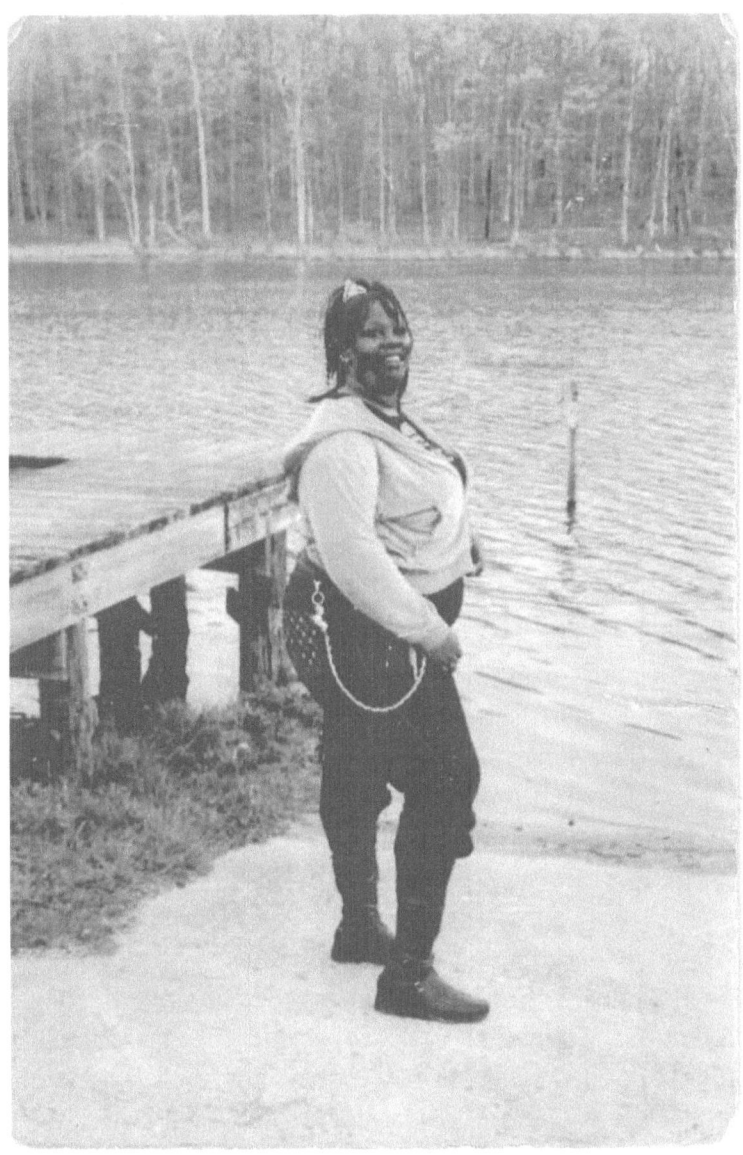

I loved the crack-cocaine high until I had to start selling my body to old men to get the money to buy it. All of a sudden, I was no longer the fresh young thing on the strip. I was now a seventeen-year-old crackhead willing to do whatever with whomever just to get the next hit. I was too well known in my community, so I had to go where the full-time prostitutes went to find tricks. There I was the new "Big Butt Bertha" on the track, and every man wanted a piece of me. I was doing okay—or so I thought—until I started getting pregnant every two or three months. In addition, I began having near-death experiences with tricks: I was almost murdered five times. Tricks would beat me up because they'd come too quickly and they'd want to come again. On some nights, they'd take me by gunpoint and knifepoint. One trick even tried to bash my head in with a cinder block. I'd give my body up quickly so as not to get killed or physically scarred for life. This lifestyle was so dangerous. Every night I prayed to God to help me get off the drugs and out of the streets.

Soon I had to change my strategy. I started dealing only with men who were short and small-framed, and even justified seniors who were seventy to eighty years old. And to find the courage to go out into the streets, I started drinking anything and everything—Cisco and Wild Irish Rose "white" were my favorites. This new method for money ended up working for a while; I met some good tricks who became my regulars. So I didn't have to walk on the track all the time anymore if a trick happened to cancel a date —maybe just once a month. My "clients" covered my financial needs, and I could comfortably continue my drug habits.

Meanwhile, my brother was trying to keep up with society's expectations. He joined Job Corps, and then graduated and found work with Metro-North. He also got himself a membership at Gold's Gym, the place for professional bodybuilders. Leroy Jr. was eighteen and doing really well for himself. He transformed his body into a fit, muscular one that the girls loved, and females just fell around him like water. In fact, he started attracting the prettiest girls in the neighborhood and even developed a few male haters because of this.

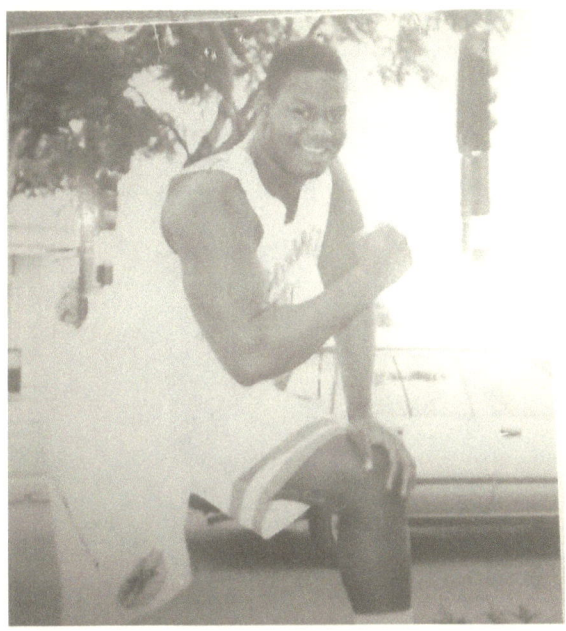

One fine day Leroy Jr. met his first love. She was light-skinned with a nice body, and for a dark-skinned brother to have a light-skinned sister, he became very popular. The two went steady for a while. Then Leroy Jr.'s girl got pregnant with his first child. When I heard the news from my street friends, I remember running around the neighborhood like a chicken with her head cut off! I was so happy that my brother was going to be a father—he'd make the greatest role model.

As for me, at eighteen I had my first baby boy, Tyshawn. By my next six-week checkup, I was already pregnant with Shayquan, my second son. But I couldn't think about being a mother—I didn't know how to be one, anyway. What I needed was to get high. Tyshawn's father hadn't been ready to become a parent, either, but regardless, we had made a baby between our drug uses. I never even knew Shayquan's father; I got pregnant while prostituting to get money to buy drugs.

Latonya R. Baskerville

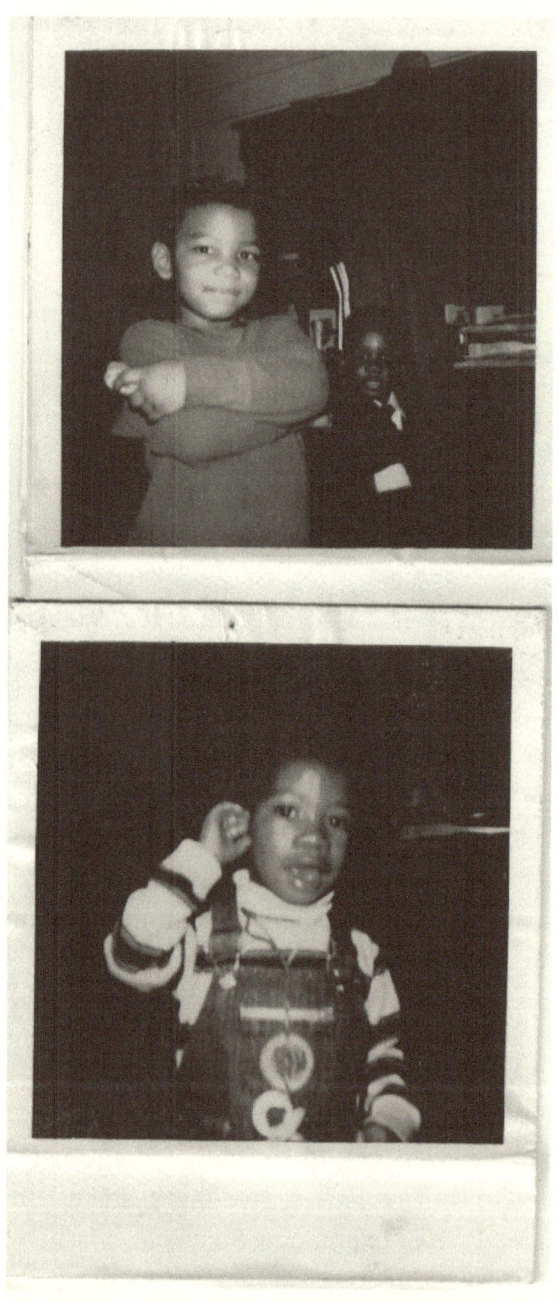

Shayquan was born with three heart chambers instead of four, and the day he was born he had heart surgery. My family didn't believe in abortions, so I continued to use drugs through every one of my pregnancies. Plus, prenatal care was too time-consuming for me, so I never attended and therefore had no idea what was going on with the baby inside me. If the baby lived, I took it to my grandma and hit the streets again. In total during this period, I was pregnant six times. Tyshawn and Shayquan lived. The others didn't.

I was twenty-three and getting high was all that mattered to me. Weed, as I recall, was my first choice because it helped me mentally cope with my insecurities. But I can't explain how crack cocaine eventually became my favorite drug. My substance abuse turned me into a straight-up junkie; I started buying anything—crack, dope, coke, weed, alcohol. You'd think that with the way I was using drugs, they'd change the way I looked. But my appearance as a six-foot-tall, 340-pound, dark-skinned woman never changed.

My self-esteem did, though. I thought I was the Sugar Honey Iced Tea when I used those drugs. It was amazing how I could still justify the ignorance of my drug abuse as crack addicts around me were shrinking like raisins and I was still big as hell with a big, fat behind. My brother was very saddened by my substance abuse. He sometimes gave me money to show his love, but he often talked to me about going into drug treatment for help. I wasn't ready to stop getting high, though, and I didn't think I had a problem with drugs. Facing rejection from society was my problem. Getting high helped me cope with it. My appearance was not going to change, and I couldn't accept that I was born this way.

One day I received a message that made me drop to my knees: Leroy Jr. was in the hospital and he was not doing well. The family was going crazy because we didn't know what had happened for him to need hospitalization. I was aware that he had many issues with his baby's mother; he had been arrested several times for his extreme handling of her. So the first thing I thought was that she had killed him this time for manhandling her.

But I was drowning so much in my substance abuse that I couldn't even stop getting high long enough to go see him at the hospital while he was being treated. Not long after he'd been admitted, my brother's rage ended up causing him to rip the IV tubes out of his body and leave the hospital. His landlord called my grandmother that day and told her that he had found my brother stretched out on the floor in a puddle of his own blood. The landlord had called 9-1-1, but from what he could see, my brother was badly suffering. Leroy Jr. was pronounced DOA by the ambulance attendant who arrived on the scene. Apparently, both his kidneys had collapsed, he had a brain tumor, and two major heart attacks had occurred before he finally died.

My family was devastated. I knew my brother had never used street drugs, though—I had given him a hit of weed one day and he had nearly choked to death. There were no hard drugs I knew of that could break a healthy young man down like that, so I started my own investigation on the streets. I questioned all my brother's friends about his hangouts and hobbies. His friends were amazed by his sudden death. Most of them didn't have any information, but one eventually came out. He said Leroy Jr. had been inquiring about the benefits of steroids. This friend had cautioned him not to mess with steroids and my brother had apparently been convinced.

But the pressure in our community during that time was very strong. Like me, my brother had also been experiencing bad feelings about his obese appearance, and had thought that a weight loss drug would be a good idea. How I wish he had asked more questions about these types of drugs and the consequences they could have. But the bullies in our community made it so hard to live in our neighborhood. Time and again, we lost all the battles. And in the end, my brother lost the fight for his life.

My Health and Addiction

I could never fully explain how I felt over the loss of my brother. We had so many good times together, and his passing left me in so much pain. Like stable, loving parents, my mom and dad had spoiled us with all the luxuries we could ask for, for nothing. Our playground was in the backyard, and I remember on many days my brother and I played there until the sun set. To this day, I still laugh when I remember how we would get in trouble because we wouldn't come in the house and bathe for dinner.

My brother's sudden death made me cry out to God and ask, "Why, Lord?" Whenever I heard songs that reminded me of him I cried until the tears ran dry. I hurt so badly, and alcohol and drugs became my salve. To keep calm, I started drinking heavily, but after a while I needed more alcohol than usual. So I would keep drinking until I blacked out. My drug tolerance had also become so high that I had to mix drugs because just one was not enough. Lethal combinations like weed and cocaine followed by liquor and beer couldn't even get me high anymore.

Using drugs was my way of numbing my low self-esteem, fear, and shame. Whenever I smoked crack, these feelings disappeared. But I would then instead become paranoid, so I mixed heroin into the crack—this was called "chasing the dragon"—then drank liquor, and the paranoia would stop.

Whenever I came off my drug binges I felt like I was starving. I ate everything in my grasp: fast foods, whole cakes, red meats, pasta, and sweets. There was a deep hole in me, and I used drugs and food to fill it. This hole became a vacuum, nearly sucking the life out of me daily.

A month later I got pregnant again and nearly died. By this point, my sixty-three-year-old grandmother was taking care of my two sons—and she just couldn't manage a third baby. My drug addiction wouldn't allow me to properly parent my children, and my grandma soon had no other choice than to report me to the Administration for Children's Services (ACS) because she needed money to take care of my kids. But I just spent the public assistance and food stamp benefits on drugs, including the Women, Infants, and Children (WIC) checks.

Shayquan's second open-heart surgery procedure was coming up soon as well. He was almost two, and his doctors had informed me that he would need another surgery around this age, because the procedure that had been performed when he was a newborn would not continue to be effective on its own. I managed to take him to most of his heart appointments and immediately rescheduled the ones I didn't attend. But ACS was not pleased with me. I was unstable and still running the streets, so they issued preventive services. An ACS worker sat down and explained to me that preventive services would give me my last chance to get my life together while my children were still in my custody. She told me that if I didn't complete preventive services, my children would be placed in foster care.

My ACS worker then referred me to an outpatient drug program. Unfortunately, at that time, I really didn't want to participate in it. I arrived late every day and drank alcohol instead of smoking crack and weed. That way, when they gave me supervised drug screens, my tests for cocaine and cannabis were always negative. I wasn't ready to stop getting high completely because I still thought I could control my drugs and not let them control me. All I needed was a better way to get high.

So instead of getting high every day, I tried to do it only on the weekends. I managed to fake my way through the drug program, but just before I was scheduled to graduate, Shayquan became ill. I called the drug program and explained my situation but was told I wouldn't graduate if I missed the last class. So my grandmother took Shayquan to the hospital while I completed class. When I got to the hospital, the doctor informed me that my baby was being admitted for tests because my little boy's heart was beating irregularly. I knew Shayquan was due for his second heart surgery, but I thought the surgery would be simple like it was when he was born. Although I was aware that it would be a serious surgery, I figured he'd still survive and then come home.

But he never came home. My baby passed away ten days later. The doctor said his heart started failing rapidly and that Shayquan was too weak to undergo surgery. My body felt so heavy when my two-year-old died—it felt like globs of meat with no bones, and my skin looked dark and ashy. Whatever was spiritually left in my body told me something was trying to kill me. I cried to God for strength and guidance through these chaotic times. I had just had a miscarriage and had buried my brother only ninety days earlier. And now this.

I couldn't endure any more. I thought killing myself would be the only way out, but I knew I would spend eternity in hell if I chose this option. In the meantime, Tyshawn was wilding out over the death of Shayquan; they had been only six months apart. He was acting out in school, starting fights, throwing chairs, hitting teachers, and stabbing children. Tyshawn's behavior was so violent that the agency wanted to place him in a group home or mental hospital. It was clear to everyone that

Tyshawn was suffering emotionally, but as a three-year-old, he didn't know how to talk about it.

This was all too much for me to handle. And I couldn't deal with the guilt that my substance abuse had caused Shayquan's death. I cried every day and torched myself with food. I ate and ate until my stomach ached. I wasn't hungry, I was hurting. Whenever I got tired of eating, I wanted to get high. My only source of money was prostitution, so I worked the streets and got more money. But I couldn't disappear for days and black out like I had before, because ACS still had Tyshawn in preventive services. ACS had the power to remove my only son from my care if I messed up and got caught. So once again, I created a plan that would let me hide the effects of the drugs from ACS and my family.

My family was so burned out by this point. They were tired of ACS' investigations into everything. One time my dad wanted to take Tyshawn for the weekend. ACS grilled my father so badly that my dad just said never mind and that he would wait until I regained custody of Tyshawn. Due to her faith in God and the power of prayer, though, my grandmother never spoke words of defeat for Satan to hear. She wouldn't ever say, "Tonya, I give up on you" or "There is no hope for you." She continued to pray for me and reminded me to pray for myself. My grandmother said the enemy was going to great lengths to destroy me, and told me God must have a grand and mighty plan for my life. She said she had only ever seen people go through struggles and trials this hard when they were the ones chosen to serve God on a very high level and win souls over to Him.

I was very pleased to hear my grandma say that because I couldn't figure out why my life was so messed up. I had lost both my brother and my son in the same year, just ninety days apart from one another. They were innocent beings who hadn't lived the way I lived. Yet their lives were cut short, whereas

I was saved many times from being murdered while prostituting. I didn't understand why God would allow such injustices to befall my family. But my Christian upbringing had taught me never to question the Holy Father.

But once again, I went right back to doing what I knew best: drinking and drugging. One night I decided to have sex with some guy with a two-letter name. He was from down South and was visiting family who happened to live in the building my grandmother managed. Three weeks later, I was pregnant. I didn't know for sure, but I figured the baby was the Southern visitor's. It didn't matter to me, though, because this was my miracle baby. The new baby was going to help me and Tyshawn heal from our loss of Shayquan.

I continued dabbling in drugs throughout my whole pregnancy. But this time, I did attend prenatal care because I wanted to make sure my baby was fully developing inside of me. Throughout the nine months I did get high, but my warped thinking told me that if I attended prenatal care, then my baby would be mentally and physically okay. Wow, drug-induced thinking is crazy!

***

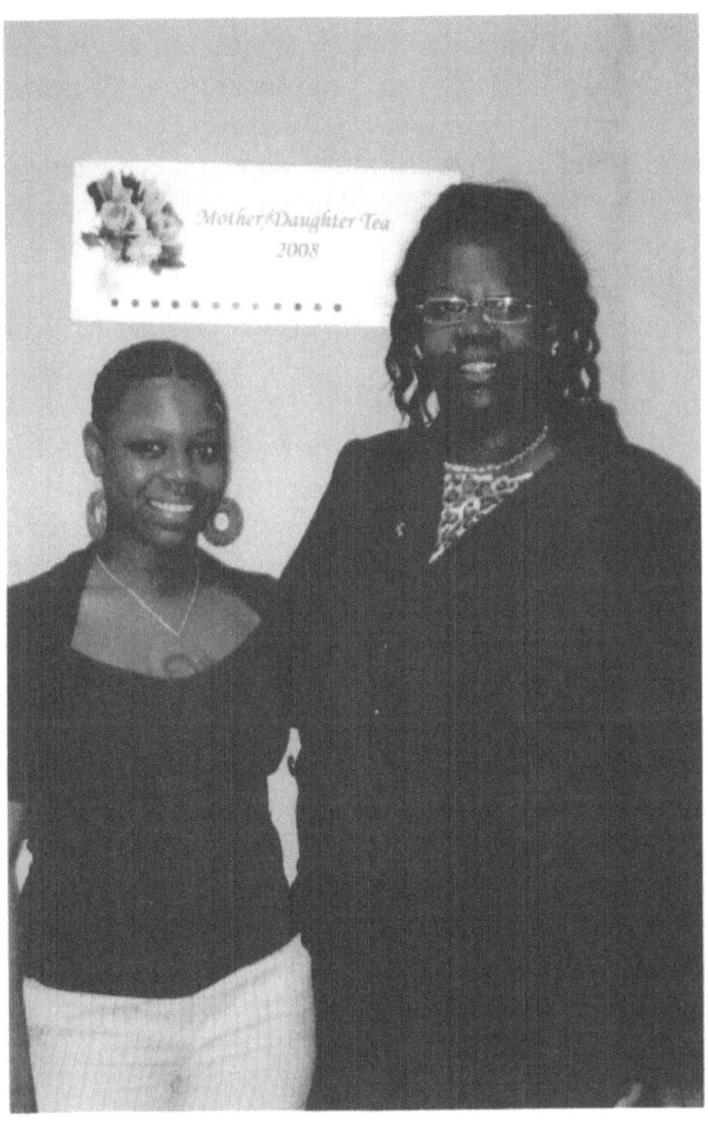

On January 29, 1993, I gave birth to a beautiful baby girl.
This made me so happy. I vowed to dress her all girlie like me
and teach her about the birds and the bees. ACS allowed me to
bring her home because they didn't know that I was still getting

23

high every now and then. If they had drug-tested my daughter, they would've found that she was positive for all drugs, especially cocaine. I wanted to control my life, but I wanted to do it my way, and I didn't give a damn about the stinking system. Even though Tyshawn wasn't in my care yet, I just knew he would be soon. All I needed to do was continue pretending to be clean and sober until I got him back. Then my nightmare would be over. And because I still wasn't ready to stop getting high, I continued to come up with better ways to do it.

So that I could be a semi-responsible parent on weekdays and a prostituting crackhead on the weekends, I practiced getting high only on weekends. I survived that way in silent suffering and pain for many years. To obtain permanent housing, I entered the shelter system with my daughter. I was still smoking crack in the shelter, but I hated feeling paranoid inside the room where me and my daughter stayed. The drugs were starting to tire me out by this point, too. They weren't giving me the same good feelings anymore. Instead, they were beating me.

But even after several years of drug use, at twenty-three, I still didn't know how to quit. Friends and family seemed to be handling their drug and alcohol issues just fine. I wondered to myself why I wasn't like them. Why couldn't I get my drink and smoke on without going to the extreme of prostituting and smoking crack? I dreamed of my life without drugs, but all I could imagine was boredom. Still, I was so tired of selling my body to smelly, old, nasty men every time I got high.

So that I could get high without any disturbance, I found an apartment in the Bronx that was far from my family. I knew they would never come all the way over from Brooklyn without calling. One day I was traveling to Brooklyn for the weekend when I met this guy on the train. He wasn't my usual bad-boy type; he seemed respectable and kind. Jay and I soon started seeing each other regularly. He took me out for dinners and movies frequently. And in 1998, I once again became pregnant.

I felt different about this pregnancy, though, because I knew my baby's father and I wasn't prostituting as often. I still weighed over three hundred pounds, so I used my weight to continue rationalizing my crack usage as well. Plus, Jay gave me money and permission to smoke crack; he wanted his first child and knew that stopping my crack usage would terminate the pregnancy. Sometimes I worried about the new law that stated all pregnant women must test for HIV and drugs. HIV was spreading widely during this time, but for some bizarre reason, my clouded mind made me more concerned about the drug tests than the HIV test. Even after all my years of prostituting for money, I wasn't at all worried about becoming infected with HIV.

When I resubmitted my blood work for my WIC recertification, I was six months pregnant. The doctor informed me of the drug and HIV tests he was doing regardless of getting my consent first. I agreed anyway, though, because I wanted to use the WIC money to smoke up. Little did I know then that the diagnosis from the HIV test would change my life forever.

When the results came back, I remember feeling like things were over for me—I cried hysterically. My doctor tried hard to calm me down and suggested I take the test again, even though he knew the results were correct. So I got retested. I prayed that the nurses had made a mistake.

My doctor then sent me to HIV counseling because if the second test were to come back positive, I would need to learn how to take care of my unborn baby. The counselor explained that there were new medical treatments that could help the baby turn out HIV-negative. So when the second test also came back positive, I was more prepared this time around and didn't cry. No, all I was focused on at that point was saving my baby.

For the first time in my life, I started thinking not about myself, but about the unborn child I was carrying inside of me.

Taking the medication was very hard in the beginning. I had to take fourteen pills a day. I felt doomed, as though my prostituting lifestyle had led me straight to death's door. There was no shot, cream, or lotion for this. HIV was called "that shit" on the streets, and if people knew you had it, your very existence was over. You wouldn't be able to walk the streets without feeling frightened or watched. It was extremely hard for me to hold my head up in my community during this time; it was like holding a boulder on a straw.

I gave birth to my third son on July 2, 1998. He tested positive for both the virus and drugs. The HIV counselor informed me that my baby would test positive for the virus during his first month, but that his own immune system would then kick in and he would test negative after the second month. ACS allowed me to take him home as long as I agreed to go into drug treatment—*again*! Of course, I agreed, but they changed their minds after a week and came to my home to remove all three of my children from my care. Apparently, ACS had reviewed my case history, which ranged back to 1989 with my deceased two-year-old. So my children were placed in Brooklyn under the kinship foster care of my grandmother. Even though I was okay with them being with my grandma, I was still very angry that ACS had changed their decision to let me keep my kids with me. Self-loathing took over my mind, and as most newly diagnosed HIV-positive people do, I told myself, "Just get high until you die." I figured that I was going to die anyway, so I might as well die getting high as I had always assumed I would. But my Lord and Savior Jesus Christ had a better plan for me.

One day I got busted making a direct drug sell to an undercover cop across the street from the public school that I lived near in the Bronx. The charge I faced was a two-felony offense; I was a first-time offender with no priors. Spending that night in jail, I remember crying and praying that if God got me out of this situation, I would never use drugs again. The next morning I was released from jail and referred to the Bronx Treatment Court the following week. Jay had heard what had happened from the neighbors in my building, so he came to the courthouse for my hearing, where the judge mandated that I attend another intense drug treatment program. But this time around, the consequences would be more harsh: jail time would be what I'd have to deal with if I didn't complete the drug program. If I did, though, the charges would be dropped and the case would be sealed.

It was now or never. I'd have to complete this drug treatment program or else do two to six years in prison and have two felonies on my record forever. I didn't see my children often; as if they were doing me a favor, ACS had granted me only two supervised visits a week for two hours each at the foster care agency. But this agency quickly allowed me to start having my visits in my grandmother's home, because the twice weekly commute to Manhattan was very hard on a sixty-three-year-old with a newborn baby. Plus, at this time, my elderly grandmother was caring for my mentally ill mother also.

When I began drug treatment, it honestly was not easy. I relived all the old feelings of rejection and pain: the divorce of my parents, the sudden death of my only brother, the illness and death of my two-year-old son, and my HIV-positive status. Drugs had turned my life into a living hell, and I couldn't even remember how it had gotten so bad. The drug treatment program became the place to find out why I thought I needed drugs to live. Soon I learned that talking about how I felt was a great alternative to using drugs. I had no problem talking about the constant rejection I experienced and how much it hurt me to be treated that way. I also tried to talk about being HIV-infected, but it was still too difficult at that time; my feelings of shame and embarrassment were still too strong. But things

were becoming clearer for me. Prostituting and having sponta-
neous unprotected sex were how I became infected in the first
place—I knew that. I had played the unprotected-sex game that
a huge percent of all humans play. And I had lost. But what I
had always been taught was, as you make your bed, so you must
also lie on it.

***

During this time, it deeply hurt me to be an African
American—I regretted that my fellow brothers and sisters were
so uneducated when it came to HIV. When someone found
out that you were positive, you were immediately treated like
garbage. People looked down on you, showing pity and sorrow
at the very sight of you, as though they were viewing your body
at a wake. In their eyes, there was no hope for you; you were
already gone.

I didn't need that kind of treatment; I needed support,
encouragement, and positivity. This would be the greatest fight
for my life. And at only twenty-eight, I was too young to be
giving up. Plus, I had to remember that my Lord and Savior had
been beaten and bruised on the cross, and had given His body
and blood to save mine. So I prayed to Jesus Christ for forgiveness and another chance, because I knew His blood heals all
sins and iniquities.[17] I started calling on my Lord and Savior
Jesus Christ and meditating on His Word every day. And He
heard me: God gave me a wonderful, loving family and true
friends to help me in my fight. There was a change that took
place in me—I became absolutely determined to survive and
continue living my life.

I believed that by every swipe Jesus took for my sins, His
blood healed me.[18] I stopped feeling ashamed of myself and
feeling that I needed to be perfect for Christ to care for me.
Never would I be perfect; I knew I would continue to make
mistakes and would always need help because I am human. I

knew God didn't afflict His children with disease, and my will became totally focused on fighting Satan with the Word of God. My faith that Jesus' blood would heal anything was all that I needed from now on. The enemy was trying to kill me because he had seen what I would do in my future in Jesus' name.[19] But I became completely determined to live for the purpose that I was predestined for.[20] No matter what diseases Satan tried to afflict me with, I was going to carry out God's will.[21]

I remembered what the pastors and my grandma had taught me about Satan: he comes to steal, kill, and destroy. And this is exactly what I had witnessed when he took away my son and brother. Their deaths had been meant to break me, and the HIV had been intended to separate me from God, kill my faith in Him, and ultimately destroy me for good. God had a plan for my life, and Satan didn't want it to happen. I became enraged with Satan for all his evil attempts. I would no longer give him my life, and dying became the last thing on my mind. Instead, I started thanking God for His grace and mercy. I prayed for long life and prosperity in Jesus' name. And my goal became to live longer than anybody I knew who wasn't infected with HIV.

My drug treatment counselors were experienced and knowledgeable regarding addiction. They knew it came in all different forms, and not just as a dependency on drugs. The effects of addiction weren't new to them, either—they had heard it all. On the day the foster care agency awarded me trial-discharge of my children, I felt like saying, "Thank you. And kiss my ass," at the discharge meeting. But I thanked them for helping me get my kids back instead. I was glad that I had stopped using drugs, and I was delighted to have successfully completed the drug program. Getting money to get high every day had been an exhausting job that had worn me down really fast at a very young age. I was finally ready to start a new chapter.

Life suddenly became worth living. I appreciated every day that I didn't have to use drugs to cope with life. My baby continued testing negative for HIV, and this made me extremely happy. After all, it had been my fault. Why should he have had to pay for my poor decisions? Soon I was referred to the Hope Program for aftercare treatment. Hope educates recovering drug addicts who are trying to build or rebuild their lives. This program also encouraged me to continue my education. This was scary for me because my reading grade was only 7.5 and my math grade was just 5.6. I thought, "How the heck am I going to complete the GED test with scores like this?"

I wasn't ready for the GED class, but I was accepted into the pre-GED program. It was hard for me to focus in class, though, because I knew my children would be coming home soon. In December 2000 they came home for good, and that year we had the best Christmas ever—we were finally all together again. I decided to postpone my GED goal until my children got settled in their new environment with me. But my substance abuse, my health status, my physical appearance, and my children's foster care experience continued to fill me with tremendous guilt and embarrassment. And for a while, I even believed that I didn't deserve the benefits of living clean because I had so many issues.

The transition for both me and my babies was tough, though. There was no aftercare training provided for families reunited from foster care. My children had been in foster care for only eighteen months, but seeing the way they behaved, you would have thought it had been eighteen *years*. Whenever they were home, I felt like a slave to their every word. No one said "thank you" to me for doing the extra things I did or showed any appreciation that I had worked so hard to reunite the family so quickly. This made me despise my children's behavior; I felt that they needed to be more grateful that I had gotten them back home.

On top of all this, I didn't know how to parent without drugs and alcohol. I was starting from scratch, essentially. By mimicking TV families, I would make unhealthy breakfasts and cook huge dinners to please my children. I baked cakes and allowed for reckless eating at any time of the day or night. My kids were given no boundaries or structure—and in terms of eating, I set no restrictions for myself, either. I spent lots of money on soul food and Chinese food. And pretty soon, I was growing bigger and bigger on a daily basis.

After a year, the same foster care agency my kids had been placed into offered me a job working with parents whose children had also entered foster care. I was terrified of leaving public assistance because it was the only financial supplement I had ever had. My former drug addiction had also weighed me down with huge insecurities and responsibilities. I really didn't think I could hold a job. And even though I was fighting to keep my life on the right track, deep down I still felt that I was going to die from HIV. Plus, at this point, I was extremely obese, had high blood pressure, and was facing diabetes. All I kept envisioning was trying to get up every morning in rain, sleet, or snow to go to work. Would I be able to do it?

My boss kept the job position open for six months because I was so afraid of becoming fully financially independent. I'd go to the foster care agency every day anyway, but I preferred the stipend as opposed to a salary. Meanwhile, my children were going through withdrawals from the foster care system; they would yell and fight with each other all the time. My household became very chaotic, but I was scared of disciplining them. All I knew was the old-fashioned way of disciplining, and I didn't feel comfortable using it. Often I'd even try bribing them with fast foods and gifts they didn't earn just to keep the peace in my home.

Soon I decided to try using the skills I had learned in drug treatment on my children. I modeled proper anger management, I put up behavior charts, and I followed proper parenting skills to the head. Birthday presents, Christmas gifts, chore rewards, allowances—everything depended on their charts. If their charts showed too much bad behavior, my kids wouldn't receive anything, regardless of the occasion. I created a parenting model to fit each child's age and cognitive ability. For example, my daughter Janera was six years old at the time and my son Tyshawn was eleven. They each needed a different parenting model because the same one wouldn't be able to work for both a boy and a girl who were five years apart. Also, because my three children all had different dads and I didn't even know two of their fathers, I had no idea if my kids were behaving like their dads or like other family members in their fathers' families. All I knew was that they were my babies and that I had to be responsible for their behavior because I had chosen to get high through all my pregnancies.

As much as I wanted to believe that getting my kids back under my care was enough, being honest with myself, I knew it wasn't. Due to my drug addiction, my children had experienced several years of neglect, maltreatment, and trauma. I didn't realize back then that my not going to school plays and events and my not taking them on family trips could cause so much emotional hardship. So they were entitled to be mad at me, and I had to learn how to accept myself for all of my past mistakes. Thank God that during drug treatment I became connected to a special group of people who promised to love me until I learned to love myself. That special group helped me accept my permanent health conditions and deal with my children's adolescent behavior with love and compassion.

But I wasn't out of the woods yet. Somehow I came to believe that I could create a family environment and solve all the problems in my household by getting married. But I went about it the wrong way, by using money to lure unprepared men into my fantasy family. I never desired educated or employed men because they would be in control of the relationship. My preference was to be with unemployable, uneducated ex-cons with felony records. You see, I wanted my men to need me as much as I needed them. I faked sexual satisfaction just so they could feel like real men whenever we were in bed together. My obesity and health status were major issues for my partners, so I paid big money to buy their love, loyalty, commitment, and trust. I was so desperate to be in a committed relationship that I even bought the wedding rings for four different men! I pretended to enjoy cooking, cleaning, and taking care of the children like a good housewife, and tried to live by the old motto that says the only way to a man's heart is through his stomach. Every day I made breakfast, lunch, and dinner for my partner. And all the while, I was growing bigger and bigger, breaking and destroying furniture everywhere I went to visit. The bigger I became, the lower my self-esteem sank.

My Guilt, Remorse, and Ultimate Triumph

Iwas only twenty-eight years old and six months pregnant when I was diagnosed with HIV, and I was scared as hell. My culture and community were uneducated on this disease, so I was subject to ignorant conversations about it every day. My own lack of knowledge was killing me slowly, so I began an emotional battle to set health goals for myself.

My first goal was to learn all I could about HIV: Where did it come from? How infectious was it really? And how many African American men and women were infected in my community? I spent over two years researching, and the things I learned amazed me.

The most highly infected groups were African Americans and Hispanics living in low-income communities. Ignorance, drugs, and alcohol played the largest part in spreading the infection. What saddened me is that the disease didn't originate in American minority communities, but these communities' rejection of education made them the most highly infected. Low-income residents were not open to learning about this disease that came from the boonies. But this virus infiltrated neighborhoods like mine like roaches and rats. Even churches criticized the virus; pastors preached that it was a curse from God. They said the people that were infected were the ones God was angry with, and that He wanted them to die like those in Sodom and Gomorrah. That lie just made things worse—it caused HIV to spread even more within communities like mine because HIV-infected members were not being truthful about their status. Instead, they were infecting as many others as possible and leaving the church. I had to do a lot of research before I gained a healthy perspective on my own HIV status.

My second goal was not to associate myself with people who were not educated on HIV. If I heard people I knew say something made up or ignorant about the virus, instead of wasting my time correcting them, I would just disconnect the relationship and "lose" their numbers on purpose. My diagnosis was enough for me to handle every day; I didn't need stupid myths and insensitive comments in addition.

Doctors and scientists have done such a fine job over the years of researching HIV and making information on it available. I'm so grateful for this, because it allowed me to empower myself with knowledge. Gradually, I learned to stop fearing HIV. I found out that blood-to-blood contact posed the highest risk of infection. I even discovered why the virus is so difficult to kill with medical treatments: HIV is an extremely smart virus. It contently mutates, so finding a cure is a very complicated process.

As I continued my research, my wisdom on HIV expanded. I learned many specifics about the virus, such as the fact that its infectiousness ranges from high to low. For example, unprotected vaginal and anal sex are considered high risk. But oral sex and saliva contact pose low risk, unless there are open sores or conditions in the mouth such as herpes and bleeding gums. That's why when practicing any kind of oral sex, your dental health must be excellent. And while the risk of infection is always there when you're practicing unprotected sex, people who are infected with HIV have a *responsibility* to inform and educate their partners before any sexual contact is made.

Ever since I had been diagnosed, my HIV status had hovered over my head like a dark, foggy cloud. Due to my status and obesity, I always accepted maltreatment and mental abuse from my partners. But despite being HIV-positive, as a single woman, I still had the desire to one day get married and complete my family. I had sexual practices that I loved and enjoyed, but I wanted to indulge in them only with the man I'd marry and commit myself to. It was a challenge to reconcile all of these emotions and desires; it's extremely difficult to handle being diagnosed with any kind of incurable illness, let alone having to deal with it all by yourself. That's why I am so glad I had my Lord and Savior Jesus Christ and my family by my side as I went through my process of struggle and healing.

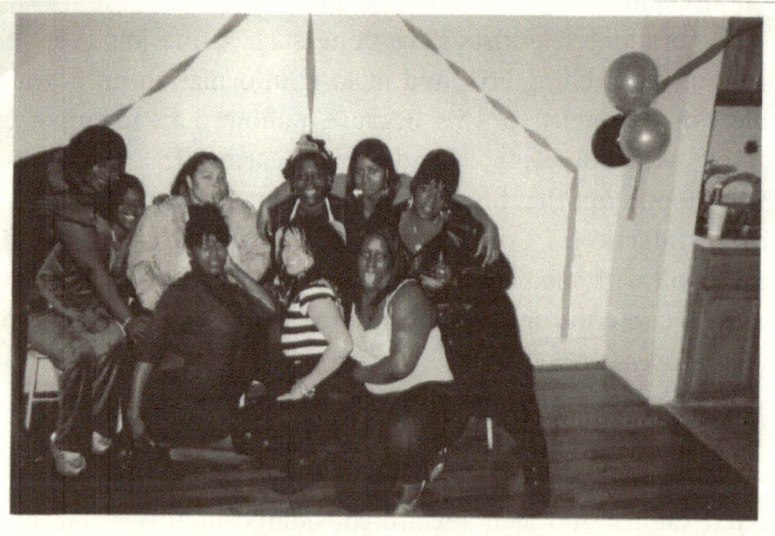

My family was so supportive and encouraging, especially my sisters and cousins. The older family members were great, too, but because I was closer in age to my sisters and cousins, their attitudes toward me were what mattered most. I never smelled ammonia and bleach around their homes when I visited. I was able to sleep in any bed I liked, even my nieces' and nephews'. I used the same bathroom and ate off the same dishes as everyone else, and was never treated like I had "that shit" or "the monster," as HIV was called in my community.

So many newly infected African American and Hispanic community members lost their battles with HIV due to the rejection they faced from their families. Most of them refused to receive an education on the deadly disease because they didn't understand it. It amazed me how many minorities refused to learn about the things they didn't understand. They didn't realize that you have to educate yourself in order to gain knowledge and understanding. The rejection and ignorance they suffered from in their low-income communities drove many angry and embittered HIV-infected individuals to go out on vicious hunts to infect others. So many people died because of this.

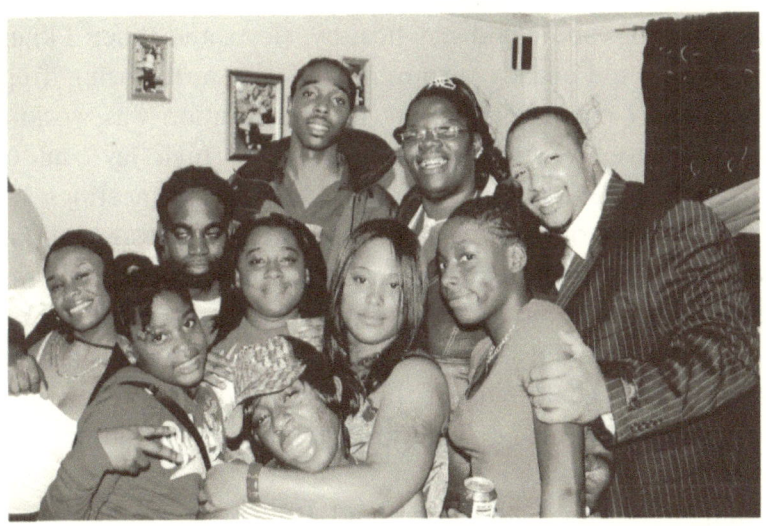

But in my family, my sisters told me, "Bitch, sit your ass down, because we are not ready for you to die.It's bad enough our brother is gone." They would walk me to my twelve-step meetings until I felt comfortable going alone. Once they saw that I had connected well with my twelve-step fellowship, my sisters became confident that I was in good hands.

My twelve-step program recommended its members to stay in our current relationships during the first year of recovery if we were in one, but if we weren't, we were encouraged not to enter a new one during our first year of sobriety. My fellow-ship also suggested that I learn about myself and the disease of addiction first, before getting involved in a long-term relationship. This was because relationships could be painful and could cause recovering addicts to relapse.

At the time, I thought I was still in a relationship with Joquan's father, Jay. We had been seeing each other since 1997 and had just recently become parents to our baby boy. But Jay never stopped getting high. And he began to find me very boring because I wasn't using drugs and having wild sex with him anymore. Regardless, I continued to attend twelve-step meetings so I could stay healthy, clean, and sober. I knew the HIV would quickly turn into AIDS if I started using drugs again, and I could tell that my HIV medication was working well, because I wasn't being tempted to get high. Jay couldn't handle this. He criticized me for attending my meetings and said they were only for weak people. Often, I'd argue with Jay, defending my twelve-step program. I had been clean for one year and my children had been returned to my care. How could I deny this program when it was making such miracles happen for me? How could I reject this special group of people who were supporting me nonstop through the highs and lows of my recovery?

But Jay was unable to understand. He started cheating on me in 2000 with a woman more suitable for his taste: she was a convicted felon who had done three years for cutting another woman up with a bottle. He had been screwing her for a year before I found out—I was so hurt. That was my first experience having to deal with my feelings without using drugs and alcohol to numb them. There was so much pain, anger, and resentment that I thought I was losing my mind. I felt a burning under my skin that I couldn't reach, so I called my cousin for advice about the situation. She simply said, "If it hurts more to keep him, then let him go." Going to my cousin's

church one day, I walked up to the pulpit and fell on the floor, crying out to God to soothe the burning under my skin. Thank the Lord, He did. After a few months, the burning stopped.

By this point in time, all three of my children were fully under my care. Tyshawn was ten, Janera was five, and Joquan was eighteen months old. It felt very strange to parent my children without the use of drugs and alcohol, and I somehow thought that having a husband would complete my family. One night, at two o'clock in the morning, I met a man during a trip I had made to a store to get Joquan a pacifier. His name was Vin.

Vin was cool, but he wasn't in recovery. He tried to stop smoking weed for me and did well for a while. But his behavior soon changed, and he became someone I didn't know anymore. The lust, anger, jealousy, deception, and envy he began displaying toward me became too much. I didn't understand why he was so angry with me for succeeding in my life.

But regardless of his behavior, I still wanted to help him. Vin dreamed of being a rap star, so I tried my best to be encouraging. But he was already thirty-seven years old, and even though I doubted his genuine interest in pursuing a future in rap, I still figured, "Who am I to decide?" I never showed my disbelief because I don't believe in discouraging anyone's dreams or plans for their life. So I went out of my way to bring Vin applications for music colleges I thought he might like to look into. But what did he do? He stuffed the applications in a drawer and continued his mission to destroy me.

In the meantime, my continued participation in their monthly parent support group made the foster care agency very proud of me, so they offered me a job making approximately $25,000 annually. This made me so happy and excited because I had never had a real job in my life. I had been on public assistance ever since I was eighteen and pregnant with Tyshawn. I had no education, work experience, or job history. My way of getting money had always been through public assistance and hustling—prostitution had been my highest-paying job. So I worked out an agreement with Vin. He babysat Joquan and put him on and took him off the school bus every day that I worked. To show my thanks and repay him, I got Vin a babysitting allowance from public assistance.

It seemed like we had created a really good family relationship, until I found out that Vin was physically abusing and starving Joquan. I started seeing suspicious scars on Joquan, and when I finally asked Vin about them, he claimed they were accidents. Let's be real: How many accidents are there that end up leaving scars on a child?! To make things worse, a sister in my building got drunk one day and told it all. The neighbors in our unit had heard everything, too, and could confirm her stories. This sister claimed that Vin had been lusting after her, telling her his most disgusting sexual fetishes. Hearing her describe them made me sick to my core. I cared a lot about Vin, but I also knew in my heart that what this woman was blabbing about was all true. And I was so embarrassed and ashamed.

Soon everybody in our neighborhood knew about Vin's freaky, repulsive sexual fetishes. I walked with my head down for months after that. And sadly, Some of my old demons returned, causing me to eat more than I should and even take up smoking—I'd light cigarette after cigarette until I was puffing three packs a day. I also again started thinking that I could find relief by killing myself through drugs or by allowing the HIV to turn into AIDS. Self-pity, guilt, and remorse consumed my body and mind. I became filled with all those negative thoughts that would no doubt take me right back to doing drugs and drinking alcohol if I didn't shake them off.

All I wanted was a companion and soul mate to grow old with, and at the time, I was still too vulnerable to realize that the kinds of men I was entering into relationships with would never treat me the way I deserved to be treated. So, gathering all my forgiveness and strength, I called Vin to see if he wanted to work things out. We had invested five years into our relationship, and I figured that it hadn't all been bad. Even though Vin had mistreated my baby, I thought that maybe because he had no kids of his own, it had been hard for him to deal with family life right out of the gate. Vin had also fairly shared his $40,000 lawsuit with me and my kids—he deserved another chance. A new environment would be the best way to make a fresh start. So I sent a request for Section 8 housing. The move was approved and I found a great apartment in Flatbush that was within walking distance from my job. I also suggested to Vin that we go to church to be baptized and start our relationship all over again. To properly prepare for marriage, we agreed to participate in marriage counseling as well.

For a while, despite some arguments, things seemed to be going okay. We had gotten baptized as a family and Vin and I were in marriage counseling. But four sessions before setting the wedding date, Vin started a stupid quarrel with me over beef franks. The next day, because I was upset, I went to work without kissing him good-bye. When I came home that evening, all of his belongings were gone. This devastated me—he had mentioned wanting to move out from time to time, but I had never seen anybody pack five years of belongings and move out in one day. He didn't leave a sock, shirt, shoe . . . Nothing. He left himself no reason to come back.

My downward cycle started all over again. I began eating myself into a state of deep sadness and pain. All I could wear now was men's clothing—that I'd have to order online—because I couldn't find women's clothes for my size and height. I was also smoking two and a half packs of cigarettes a day, until I started coughing up blood. This brought me to the hospital with terrible chest pains. I was convinced I had lung cancer.

Thank God for the blood of Jesus because it turned out to be only a throat infection. I took the antibiotic I had been prescribed, and after eight days, I was okay. The shame, guilt, embarrassment, and self-pity I was hiding had to be exposed because I was finding ways to try to kill myself even without drugs and alcohol. In September 2004, I accepted Vin's decision to break up with me. I didn't crawl on my knees and beg him to stay like I had before. After all, he had mistreated my baby because he had been angry with my accomplishments. He apologized to my children for his actions and we all forgave him. But I knew his feelings would resurface and interfere again if we were to continue our relationship; my success would never be something he could handle. So I respected his decision to leave. I was truly grateful for all his help and thankful he stayed as long as he did, but going our separate ways really was the best thing for all of us.

To find my strength again, I started praying to my Lord and Savior Jesus Christ every day. I promised God I was going to practice coming to Him more often about my feelings regarding my HIV status, my physical appearance, and my loneliness. I asked Jesus Christ to forgive all my mistakes and begged Him to keep the cigarettes away. And on November 16, 2004, I stopped smoking. My experience coughing up blood had scared the hell out of me. Plus, I still desired a good relationship with a real man and didn't want smelly cigarettes to interfere. Once again, my Lord and Savior had helped me get back on track. I was starting to see things more clearly now in terms of what I deserved in a relationship, too. In all honesty, who wants to be stuck in a marriage with a spouse who is envious and jealous of you? I didn't want to be sleeping with my hater.

I soon went back to the comfort of my twelve-step fellowship and told them what had happened. They hugged me and welcomed me back without casting judgment or asking questions. It felt so good to be back with my fellowship again. And after what I had endured with Jay and Vin, I now felt I needed a sponsor as well. But I didn't feel comfortable with women. Although I'm a strong advocate for women, my past experiences with other females had taught me that I shouldn't mingle with or trust them. So I adopted a brother in my fellowship named Jeffin as my intern-sponsor.

Listening to Jeffin's story of his cheating spouse was something I could relate to. We had both experienced disloyalty from our significant others, so I felt we had a lot in common and soon began fantasizing about us getting together. I followed Jeffin around to our twelve-step meetings in the hope of starting a concrete relationship with him and even purchased him things to try to influence his decision to get with me. But what I neglected was the fact that Jeffin had been married for over ten years. He often talked enthusiastically about starting over, but he really loved his wife and couldn't let her go, regardless of her mistakes. I couldn't blame him; I would have fought to save my marriage, too. Still, I wanted so much for a good man to love me, and Jeffin seemed just right.

After a while I became tired of being dragged along, so I gave Jeffin a choice: get with it or forget it. Jeffin wasn't ready, but my financial influence was extremely strong, so we decided to start a little something. Six months into it, though, his wife got word and called him back to her. When he broke the news to me, I was quite upset. But I didn't bother to fight Jeffin's decision to go. At this point, I was mentally worn out and so very tired of purchasing relationships with men who didn't want me.

I had been broken into tiny pieces, and I wanted badly to heal. So I kept an eye out for another male sponsor to help me process all these dysfunctional relationships. In February 2005, I asked a program member named Dupree to sponsor me. Dupree was a very handsome OG from the hood, and he was also very firm and kind. On meeting him, though, I reflected on the men from my past. Somehow, I was totally incapable of choosing the right kind. So this time, I decided only to let Dupree know how handsome I thought he was and nothing else!

Dupree and I spent a lot of time doing twelve-step work that I needed in order to discover what my defects were. During this time, I learned so much about myself and my inner motives. I realized I was searching for a man who would love and nurture me like my dad had, even though the men I chose were nothing like my father—my dad was a hard worker and would never have accepted money from a woman with children.

But my HIV status distorted my choice of men. I still recall Vin often saying that I should have felt lucky he was with me because I had *that*. Well, I would tell him to kiss my ass because I don't have *that*, I *live* with that. From the get-go, I always let men know of my HIV status. I believed that I should give them a choice right away so there would be no surprises for either one of us. The key to my health was always to be true to myself first, and then to others. So I was never angry about my status, nor did I ever want to infect others out of spite. I took responsibility for my past indiscretions as well as their consequences.

I am so grateful to my Lord and Savior Jesus Christ that my children were not born with HIV. But I know there are many children born with HIV whose parents are dead, dying, or still getting high while hoping to die. My goal is to help those children. I want to teach them how to accept their situations and live happily, healthily, and honestly. And I want them to know that having pity as a partner will not allow them to live productive lives. It's one thing to know that your lifestyle choices are what led to your infection, and another thing entirely to be born infected without having had any other choice. The pain and anger of being born HIV-positive are unexplainable. But as someone who later contracted HIV, I still had to fight to develop a strong desire to live, no matter what. This determination is what I want to pass on to others.

***

As I continued my process of healing and self-discovery, I started attending clean and sober parties because they played music I love. One night at one of these parties, as I was dancing my butt off, I glanced at the exit and there he was: the man I wanted to marry! He was my sweet flavor—tall, dark, and extremely handsome. He wore a maroon outfit with a fitted hat to match, and I thought he was gorgeous. I just had to have a taste of that chocolate! Just to make sure this brother was as handsome as it seemed, I followed him into the buffet room where the lights were brighter. Well, to my delight, he was still fine as hell, and because he had seen me following him, he came over to me and whispered an erotic statement into my ear. I smiled and then responded with my own erotic reply. And before I knew it, I was caught up with yet another man.

His name was Larry. He said my response was cute and sexy and that he wanted to get to know me better, so we exchanged numbers and agreed to meet again at the next party. We both couldn't wait to see each other again, and I knew I'd have to look irresistible. So at that next party, I wore a fitted spandex jean suit that revealed every curve. When I saw Larry walk in, my face lit up like a Christmas tree. He was also obviously very pleased with what he saw. He walked over to me and whispered, "Let's go to my house in Queens and get to know each other better." So we left the party, jumped in my 1983 Ford Tempo, and drove to his place. Once we got there, though, I realized it was probably still too soon to be going into this man's home. But out of curiosity, I accepted his invitation anyway and allowed him to take me.

When we finished, I remember feeling as though I loved him even though I didn't really know him yet. Larry's sex game was off the chain, and that's where I got stuck. He handled me with so much nurture and care. My size had always given men the impression that I needed tough and rough sex, but what I actually needed was tenderness. Larry's gentle sexual affection made me feel as though he loved me, so we started having sex regularly. After a while, though, I wanted to know more about him. But Larry wouldn't talk to me. He'd just come to my house, say hello, and we'd move right on to having sex. So I started complaining to him about wanting to spend a night out or go to a movie—something. And once again, I fell into old patterns: I tried to buy Larry's love, commitment, and trust. But he refused the money; he said he wouldn't take money from a woman with children and told me to buy my kids something with my money instead.

Larry didn't want a real relationship with me, though. He just enjoyed having sex—every call was for sex. But soon his regular weekly calls turned into biweekly calls. Then the calls became monthly. After a while, Larry stopped calling altogether. I felt abandoned, lost, and completely confused, so I went looking for him. I started asking people about his whereabouts and usual hangout times. When I finally found him, he wasn't happy to see me at all. It had made him upset and angry that I had been looking for him. But I persisted, telling him that I at least needed closure if whatever we had going was over. Larry didn't ever say the actual words to me, but his actions made it quite clear that we were done.

I cried like a baby night after night over Larry for months and months; I didn't want to let him go. My son Tyshawn reminded me that men don't terminate relationships with good women, and that I just needed to let it go. In addition, Dupree told me that if I continued to hold on to my relationship with Larry when I shouldn't, I wouldn't be pulled, I'd be dragged. I was tired of being dumped, so I tried to let Larry go by replacing him with a hobby.

There was a pool table in the place where Larry hung out. In my frame of mind back then, of course, I had to start playing pool where I knew I would see him. So every day after work, I went to the poolroom. With time and practice, I actually became a very good pool player, beating some of the local pool sharks who played there. A brother even congratulated me on my commitment to playing pool and gave me a brand new pool stick. This made me so happy, and it was a much-needed boost for my confidence. Playing pool became my means of relaxation. It gave me something positive to look forward to and get better at doing. Larry's abandonment and rejection of me were no longer what I concentrated on. I looked at him like a stranger now, and I even embraced his new girlfriend, Maria, who was actually very nice. Even though I still did desire a male companion, finding one wasn't as urgent for me anymore.

One night I met a pool player name Caesar. Caesar loved having intimate relationships with extremely young girls. But I still found myself enjoying our conversations, which soothed my wounds from my past four relationships. Caesar and I exchanged phone numbers at one point, and then he sent me home in a taxi. Although some people said he was a fat, broke-back pimp with not one good thing in him, I found Caesar very charming. What I should have done right then and there is run back to my twelve-step fellowship for comfort and healing after Larry rejected me. But instead I started hanging out in the drug-infested pool hall, following Larry around and passing my time with Caesar. Whereas Larry and I had met in the fellowship, Caesar was not a member of it—he drank alcohol and smoked weed. But despite his questionable reputation and habits, I had lots of fun with him; he knew how to make me laugh. I was still in a great deal of emotional pain, and Caesar seemed to calm and heal it. He did things with me that I had never experienced while growing up. Whenever we went to the movies, arcades, and Coney Island, Caesar made me feel like a teenage girl who was with her boyfriend.

A person makes the worst mistakes when in rebound mode, and that's exactly the place I was in. Not being able to think straight, I found myself developing strong feelings for Caesar and soon let him know. I told him about my health status because I wanted to be true with him and give him a choice. He had concerns but was grateful for my honesty, saying that if more infected people would share their HIV status, the rate of infection wouldn't be so high in low-income communities. His thoughts made total sense to me, as I, too, believed that my life and well-being depended on my partners' safety. Prior to becoming infected, I hadn't been responsible or knowledgeable enough to demand condom usage. But I also hadn't purposely chosen to get HIV.

Caesar stated that he didn't like rushing into sex. He believed it would distort the relationship, and he liked getting to know a woman before having sex with her. So we spent days and nights talking. All of this made being with Caesar so different from my experiences with other men. He taught me how to recognize when a man really wants a relationship. Men who only want sex, he said, won't wait too long for it. But if a man seriously wants a relationship with a woman, he will wait. The two of us laughed and played all the time, and I found that I really enjoyed Caesar's company, humor, and companionship. We finally agreed to start having sex one year into our relationship. Things were looking good for us.

As time went on, I received a settlement for $15,000 from the Section 8 Family Self-Sufficiency Program I had completed in 2007. Caesar was driving a 1995 Cali at that point, and he often complained that his legs ached and that he wished he had a truck. If I knew then what I know now, I would have just told him to lose weight, but I was none the wiser. So instead, I pulled a few strings to get my money quickly, and then I offered him $2,000 to help him buy a truck. Thanking me, he asked whether he could borrow an extra $3,000. He promised he would pay me back every penny, claiming that he had all these construction jobs lined up. Supposedly, he and his partner Kalvin were doing well in the construction business. Well, my grandmother had raised her babies to share with anybody if they could, and this is also exactly what Jesus says to do in the Bible. So I loaned Caesar the additional $3,000. I never created a payment promissory note because he was my man, and his word was good enough for me.

Soon afterward, Caesar called his daughter Wanda in Virginia and asked her to look for a nice truck for him. Within a month, she had found Caesar a very nice ride and drove it to New York for him. In exchange, Caesar gave me his Cali. I didn't know his car needed a new transmission until it started breaking down and leaving me stranded in the street, so I purchased a refurbished transmission after having a friend do an inspection. This was only the beginning of my troubles with Caesar.

In the meantime, I had seen Larry a few times and he hadn't looked the same. The word on the streets was that he had started using drugs again. I felt terrible. I really missed Larry, but he wouldn't let me inside of him. We were from the same twelve-step family and were more alike than we were different. So I would have welcomed Larry back into my heart immediately, even if we weren't a couple. At the same time, though, I knew that I couldn't keep dwelling on Larry and all my past mistakes; I had to move forward and see what the future held.

Caesar and I were planning to have sex for the first time in the Bahamas under the moonlight. December 16, 2006, was our commitment date, and we celebrated every month on the sixteenth. Caesar's birthday was also in December, so we were going to be celebrating that occasion as well as our one-year anniversary in the tropics. At this time, I was still working for the foster care agency and making really good money. So I made the reservations for our flight to the Bahamas and for our hotel accommodations. I paid for the trip in full and made sure we were all set. But just as I had started preparing passport information for us, Caesar ran into some big trouble. I received a phone call from a girl name Mina one day. She said she was Caesar's niece and told me that he had gotten arrested. I asked Mina what had happened, but she said she didn't know. So I thanked her for informing me and told her to let Caesar know that I was going to find out what had happened.

The next person I heard from was Caesar's sister Dorothy. She called me to say that Caesar and his construction partner Kalvin were being held at Brooklyn House for extortion. This made me extremely upset. We were only two months away from traveling to the Bahamas, and I had paid an unrefundable total of $2,500 for that trip. I started praying for the patience and tolerance to go through this with Caesar. Then one night I received a three-way call from Mina and Caesar. Caesar said that he and his partner Kalvin had been set up by the construction task force. He told me that he needed a lawyer because of his criminal background—a legal aid wouldn't be enough. So I started searching for an attorney. I even called Johnny Cochran's firm, which wanted $50,000 to start. That wasn't in any way possible for me to afford, so I declined and continued searching. Finally, I found a cost-efficient attorney who agreed to take the case. He wanted $2,500 up front, so Wanda and I gave it to him. The case was very exhausting and very expensive. I even took it upon myself to go to the attorney's office to see the evidence the DA had on Caesar and Kalvin. When I got there, it seemed to me as though they were intimidating the man. The situation just didn't look good at all.

We fought the case for a year and a half. It ended up being extremely expensive because the attorney wanted approximately $1,200 every other month. The money I was making at work was barely enough to maintain my family and take care of my household responsibilities. So I started talking to Caesar about making a deal with the DA and to get the case over with. Being stubborn and unwise, Caesar acted like he didn't have a long criminal history. But after six months, he agreed to cut a deal: he was sentenced to one and a half to three years in jail.

Aside from all this drama, Caesar's niece Mina was still staying at Caesar's apartment. But she wasn't paying rent, so the landlord had started the eviction process. I spoke to the landlord about holding the apartment, but she said she couldn't and that the apartment needed to be vacated. So I contacted my prepaid legal attorney, who stated that Caesar's apartment couldn't be evicted as long as the rent was being paid every month.

I spoke to Mina about this. The girl was only seventeen and couldn't hold a public assistance case open longer than thirty days. Mina also had a three-year-old daughter, so I knew she would need some help and support. Caesar asked me to take care of her and I did. I took her food shopping and called her to make sure she was okay. We were getting along fine, soon talking for hours at a time. But suddenly she started acting funny whenever I would talk about my love for Caesar. Caesar would then call up angrily, asking me what I had done to upset Mina. I'd tell him, "I said nothing to offend her. All I did was talk about my love for you." So he recommended that I don't talk to her about him anymore.

As time went on, Mina started losing her cool. She repeatedly became very angry with Caesar and at one point took the rent money that Kalvin had given her and spent all of it. This made

Caesar's landlord furious: he was now $4,000 in arrears on rent. Soon Caesar's behavior changed, too. He would call Mina and talk softly to her, often insulting me to make her laugh. This satisfied her immensely. She would laugh for hours at all the mean and hurtful names Caesar would call me. Needless to say, I didn't find the insults funny in any way. I was saddened and hurt that he would make such nasty comments about me just to entertain another female. So I started taking steps of my own. I stopped allowing the three-way calling and connected my own phone to the correctional facility.

Regardless of his disrespect toward me, I maintained my civility. I even tried to save Caesar's apartment for Mina and her daughter until Caesar came back home. So one day, I called the landlord, advocating for the apartment. She was angry and unwilling to listen to me or cooperate. She screamed, stating that she was tired of Caesar's games and wanted the apartment. Her outburst frustrated and angered me, so I decided to go to the management office and speak to the landlord's supervisor. The landlord's disrespect was not something I would just allow myself to accept. I had never even met the woman, but she needed to know that I was not just some ghetto chick who wanted to meet her outside with my Vaseline and sneakers! No, we'd do things the real way. What I wanted was to meet the company she worked for in court.

When I got to the management office, the landlord's mannerisms became totally different—she was much more receptive and respectful. She even apologized for her outburst, explaining that Caesar had caused trouble in her building in the past and that she was tired of him. Going to meet the landlord in person turned out to be important for another reason, too. As we talked that day, the landlord shared information with me about Mina and her real relationship with Caesar. What I heard upset me tremendously, and when I went home, I immediately gave Mina a call.

I got right to the point, begging her to tell me who she was to Caesar. But she continued to claim that Caesar was her uncle and that he had been helping her with her daughter because her father had died. I inquired about how long she had known Caesar. Mina claimed about three years. I then asked her where her mother was, but Mina never answered that question. Just then, my phone rang—it was Caesar. When I asked him about Mina, he told me that she was not his blood relative but a family friend. This is could believe; I have family friends who are bonded to me in the same way. So, out of love and respect, I decided to take Caesar's word for it.

By this point, I was financially struggling because I was taking care of Mina and visiting Caesar every weekend. Each trip upstate cost $150: the stay was always six hours long and there was no other choice than to eat from the vending machines. I didn't have food stamps and no one was helping me support Caesar. Caesar claimed that his friends would pitch in money for him, but, of course, they never did. Whenever I would call his friends to confirm the money they were supposed to lend, their phone numbers would mysteriously have been changed. Caesar assured me that once he came home he would help me get back on my feet and pay me back the money I spent on him. He thanked me for being so loving and supportive to him and Mina. It was the least he could do—I suffered for two years under financial distress, often neglecting to take care of my own rent, my children's needs, and my other bills.

The Mina caper finally came to a head one day when it was revealed that she wasn't Caesar's family friend at all. She was in fact Caesar's underage girlfriend. This brought me to my knees. I ran back to my twelve-step fellowship, crying and shaking from all the bullshit I had gone through for Caesar. I admitted to my twelve-step family the error of my ways. And I shared how hurt I was by the betrayal and dishonesty I had experienced for two whole years, all because of Caesar and Mina.

A brother from my twelve-step family gave me a big hug that day. He said he was very touched by my story, offered his help, and asked for my phone number. I was more than happy to reconnect with my fellowship. I felt like I was a part of the family again. It was what I should have been doing all along, even before I got into this mess with Caesar. For so long, I had stopped going to meetings because I had been too busy traveling upstate to visit Caesar every weekend. So I started meeting regularly at twelve-step sessions with the brother who had offered his support to me. He soon became my "bestie," a friend I could talk to about whatever I wanted.

So here I was, in complete financial disarray. I was $5,000 in arrears on rent and had five unpaid parking tickets. Caesar made it really hard to function, because everything was always a crisis for him. Still, I catered to his every whim. But I had never done a jail bid before, so I didn't know how to tell him that I didn't have any more money. Caesar dragged me into what I believed was the most stressful and reckless relationship I had ever been in. To work through this pain, I spoke to my bestie every day. He even started coming to my house to spend time with me. We would watch movies, talk, laugh, and play. But I was never ever unfaithful to Caesar with my bestie, because I still loved Caesar and wanted to be with him once he came home. Caesar claimed Mina was a jealous ex whom he was in debt with. He swore he had nothing more to do with her and that she just wouldn't leave him alone. These were all lies, of course. But despite my gut feeling, I believed him. I was vulnerable and my head wasn't in the right place at the time. Being alone scared me, and Caesar filled a large space in my heart by giving me laughter, joy, and companionship. I loved him so much that I even added him to my housing voucher and found an apartment in Bed-Stuy, just as he had requested.

I should have known that the more I did for Caesar, the more he'd continue to take from me. Starting the very day Caesar came home, he'd run the streets, stay out all night, and never call. I was reaching my limit with him. We argued about his nightly activities, but he didn't want to change. Soon he started bringing his little daughters to spend nights with us. These girls were five and eight, and it didn't take long at all for me to fall in love with them. Plus, they kept my mind off of Caesar's night life. But despite everything he did to try to change my mind, I became really tired of talking to him about staying out all night. It soon occurred to me that he was going to do whatever he wanted, no matter how I felt about it.

After planning it and waiting for so long, Caesar and I also finally had sex—and let me tell you, he was horrible. He was afraid of me due to my HIV status, and I'm convinced he had sex with me only to shut me up. I hated this experience with Caesar: it was fast and sloppy, and this was not what I had expected after waiting for two whole years. Caesar's preference was to have unprotected sex with fifteen- and sixteen-year-old girls. This man was in his late fifties and I was in my late thirties. As much as I had hoped he'd change, I knew I could never satisfy Caesar's fetish to sleep with children.

One day I smelled an unhealthy scent on Caesar and it turned my stomach. I remembered smelling the same scent on Mina one evening when we were writing letters to the board on Caesar's behalf. When I called him out on it, Caesar decided to move out of my house. This time, I totally agreed with no hesitation. We needed space from each other. Once he was gone, he claimed he was renting a single room in Queens from his friend and called me daily to keep his scam going, which, at the time, I was still too naïve to recognize. Just so he could keep in contact with me, I even purchased Caesar a $400 BlackBerry phone. But gradually, I began to wonder why Caesar never invited me to his so-called new home.

One evening Caesar texted me to ask about my children. When I responded, the message that I got back was the straw that broke the camel's back. The text I received said, "Don't call or text Caesar no more. He don't want you. The only kid he has is with me. By the way, this is Mina." I was shocked! I responded, "Mina the niece?!" It was so messed up. To top things off, my Cali was towed off my block from right in front of my house because I couldn't pay my parking tickets. It had kept breaking down anyway, though, so I didn't even bother to get it back. And I really didn't want any reminders of Caesar around me anymore.

I wondered why Caesar and Mina had wanted to hurt me so badly. What did I do to deserve being scammed like this? This experience was the absolute end to my dealing with men who were not a part of my twelve-step fellowship. As I had so many times before, I went back to my twelve-step family beaten, broken, bankrupt, and hurting. It seemed that each one of my relationships had left me feeling worse than the last. Once more I cried out to God to please help me forgive every single man that had hurt me.[22] No matter what they had done to me or how much it had cost me, there was no getting around not forgiving them; my relationship with God was at stake.[23]

My intent was never to hurt or kill any of my partners with my HIV. I was always truthful about my status right from the start, before engaging in any kind of sexual contact. So what was I doing wrong? These men had all dumped me without giving warning or any indication that they wanted to leave. I would have accepted the termination of our relationships without showing any malice or displaying inappropriate behavior. There was no deep-rooted hatred I felt toward men—in fact, all the men whom I'd grown up with in my life had been good to me, even the men who had married into my family. The only thing I could assume was that the men I got involved with didn't find it easy to leave the comfort of what I could provide them financially.

I am grateful to God that I didn't become a wounded female on a mission to destroy every man I met. Yes, I lost thousands of dollars that I should have used to pay off my personal debts. Yes, I made the mistake of trying to purchase love, loyalty, commitment, and trust by buying my partners any and every material thing they asked for or wanted. It didn't matter to me that I was in debt up to my neck. My feelings about my HIV status and my weight caused an overwhelming sense of guilt and desperation, a lack of proper self-respect, and an extreme fear of rejection. It just didn't seem possible that a man could sincerely love me when I had all these issues.

Though I never used hard drugs again, buying love, loyalty, commitment, and trust ended up costing me more than crack ever did. I was ashamed and embarrassed that after everything I'd done for happiness, all it had brought me were debt and loneliness. At this point, I didn't think about using drugs or alcohol; I just didn't want to be homeless. My previous partners had moved on to women more suitable for their tastes, all my money was gone, and I was tired of falling over and over again into a cycle of emotional eating. I didn't realize it then, but I know now that my food binges were putting me on the brink of eating myself to death. I would bake a whole cake and eat it alone along with a pint of ice cream every single night. Chinese food and fast food served as the appetizers before my main meals. And McDonald's Everyday Value Meals were my snacks between ten and eleven each night.

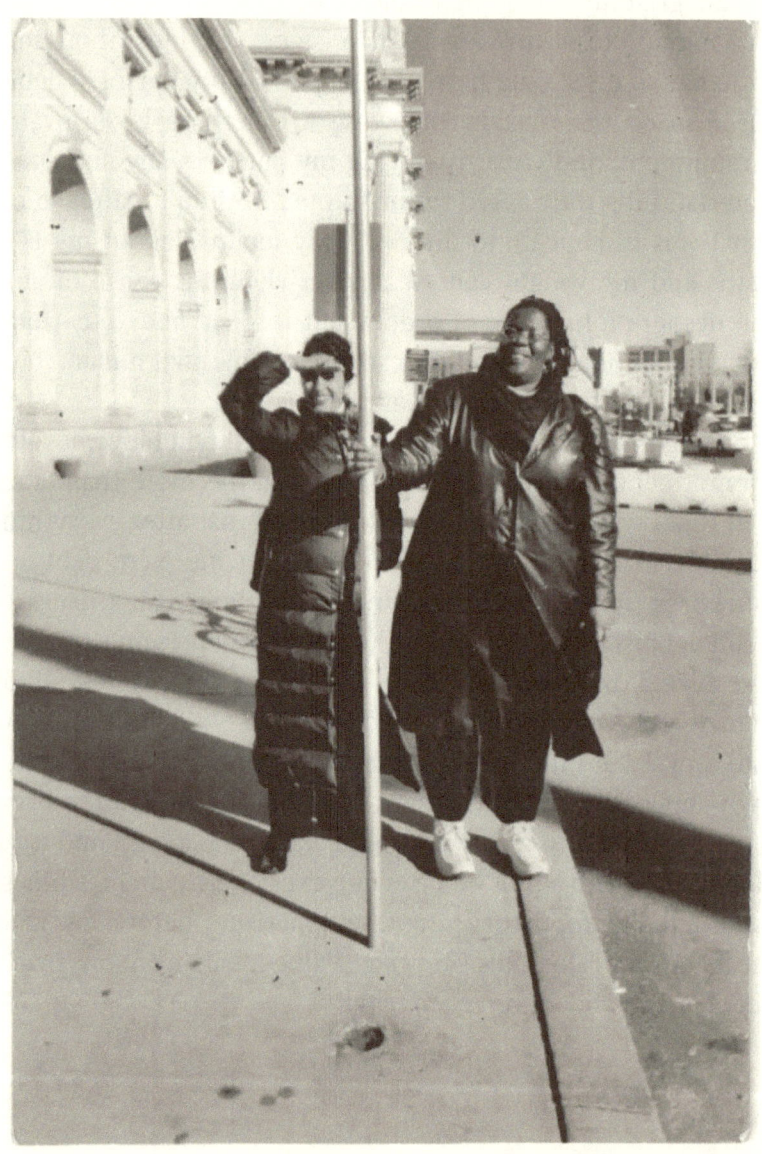

So many nights I cried. An addiction to food replaced my previous addictions, and if I had left it unchecked, it would have finished the drugs' and alcohol's job of killing me. My weight and height had by this point made it very difficult for me to sit and stand—I couldn't sit without flopping down, nor could I get back up once I sat. I had reached a stage where my bones couldn't support my weight anymore, and my legs ached every day. One day I found myself not being able to get off the toilet due to my weight; my legs had become locked in the sitting position. I called for my son Joquan to help me off the toilet. The expression on his face pushed me to a turning point. I simply had to do something about my weight.

I didn't have money to join a gym or purchase special food. I couldn't even feed my children properly because of all the debt I was in. So I went to a local sneaker store and told them my problem. The people who worked there suggested a cost-efficient pair of sneakers that would help me start my mission. My first walk was along Avenue D and Flatbush to Prospect Park, around the outskirts of the park, and then back to Avenue D and Flatbush. Oh, my God! That was about six miles, and I was in so much pain. All night I moaned like a wounded animal. But all I had to do to keep myself motivated was remember the look on my son's face as he had helped me off the toilet.

Every single day for a whole year I walked. About thirty days after my first walk, I stopped aching. A transformation was happening for me. I started feeling great after my walks and developed an overwhelming desire to accept my health issues. My substance abuse had influenced my HIV status, but that was part of a past I couldn't change. And I couldn't keep living in the past. What was done was done, and no matter what, I realized, God would have the final say.

My beginning and my end are in His hands.[24] Jesus has custody of us due to the shedding of His blood.[25] Diseases and plagues are none but tools of Satan to kill, steal, and destroy those who have faith in God. Faith is the foundation for a prosperous life.[26] And Satan wanted me to believe that a new life would be impossible for me to achieve. He is a liar.[27] I rebuke his thoughts and his fears.[28] And I enjoy my new life in Jesus Christ's name, no matter what!

PART II

My Inspiration

I often found the inspiration to continue my mission to lose weight whenever my children hugged me and expressed their pride in me. They enjoyed telling their friends about our victories over the struggles of our life together. It empowered them . . . And this, in turn, empowered me. My kids provided me with so much support during this phase of my life. It has been one of my greatest blessings.

As I achieved a healthier weight, my childhood friends could hardly recognize me—they would have to do a double take just to confirm my identity. I began receiving compliments by the dozen every single day. And suddenly, I could understand the overwhelming joy my brother must have felt once he transformed his own body and began receiving attention from girls: On seeing the change in my appearance, every one of my ex-boyfriends was amazed at my new shape. They couldn't help but let their mouths hit the floor.

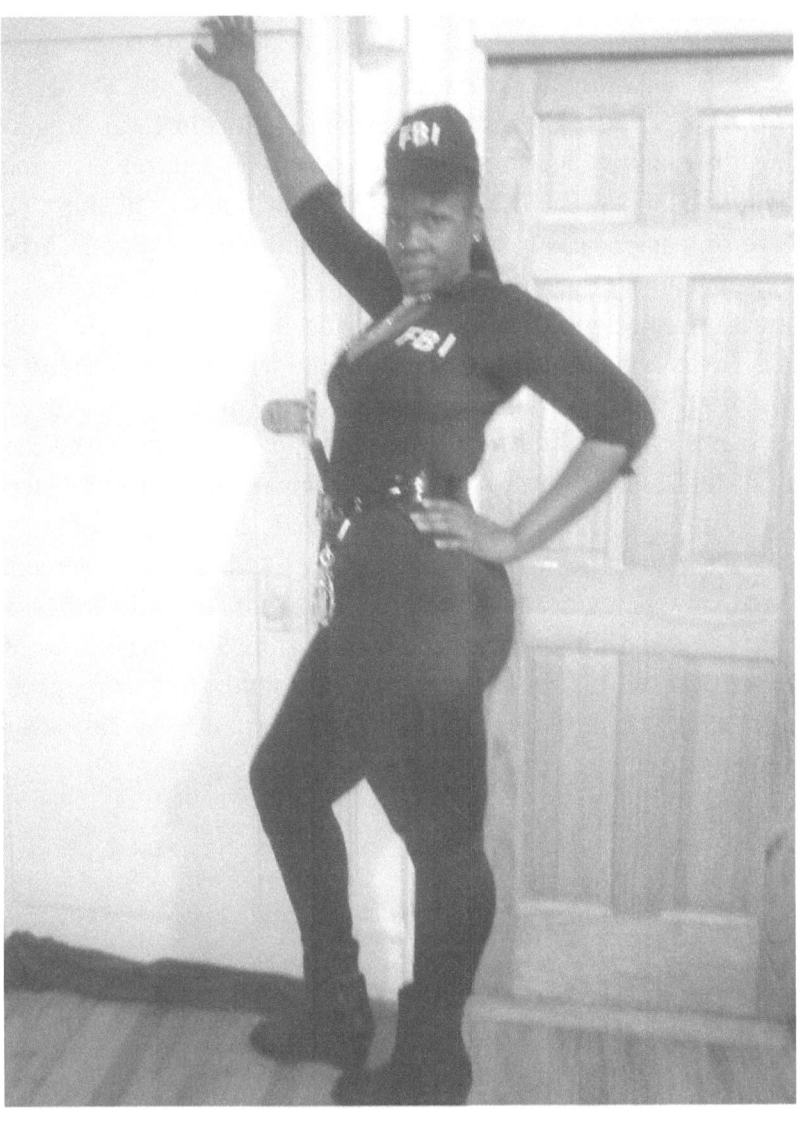

One day I was passing out flyers for a local official when I ran into Larry. My heart stopped; I had thought that I would never see him again. We hugged and my whole body started throbbing. Larry had gotten word on the streets of how Caesar had mistreated me. He expressed his deepest sorrows and said he felt partially responsible because I had met Caesar while looking for him. Then Larry grabbed me in his arms and said that I was a good woman, and that he loved me and would never let anybody hurt me again.

When Larry said those words to me, I thought I was dreaming. In a state of complete shock, I called Dupree. Dupree congratulated me and reassured me that I deserved the true love of a man because, yes, I am a good woman. Soon Larry began calling me every day. He was now in drug treatment and looking really good. He was enjoying his drug-free life with me. Every time we made love I knew he was not going to leave his drug-free lifestyle again. Larry began opening himself up to me, and we would talk about anything that was bothering him. I told him that the spiritual principals of my twelve-step program were what had kept me clean, sober, and able to survive my emotions without the use of drugs and alcohol. Gradually, Larry accepted responsibility for his actions in his own life and decided to surrender everything else to God. Once he completed his drug treatment, he found an apartment at a walking distance from mine. We've been side by side ever since.

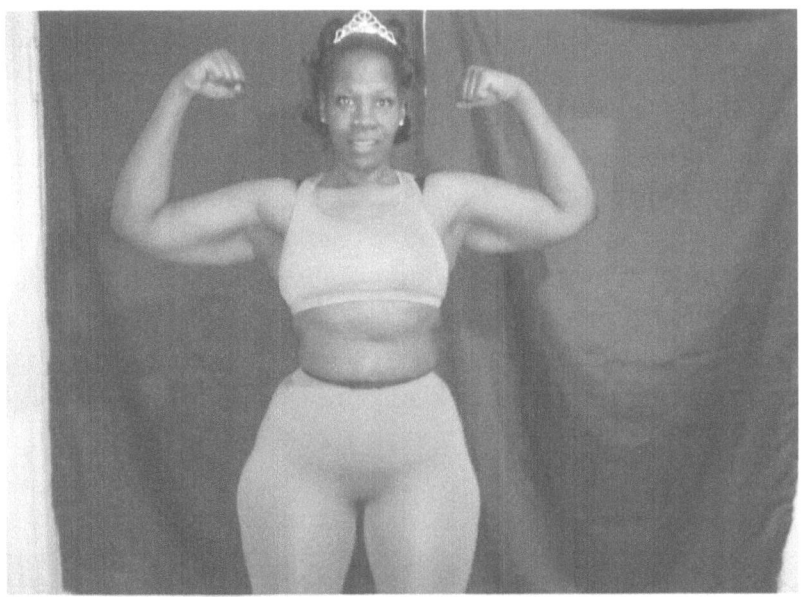

By this point, I had lost 130 pounds* and had been able to keep the weight off for over two and a half years. But all of a sudden, my health took a drastic turn for the worse: I began having pelvic spasms. For over six months, I was in constant pain, unable to work because the spasms would happen on public transportation and in clients' homes. Pain medication was prescribed for me until my dosage exceeded two thousand milligrams a day. So I went to my doctor and was soon referred to a rectal surgeon.

After examining me, the surgeon informed me that the only remedy for my pain would be to perform an operation that would permanently remove the muscles causing my spasms. But this would affect my ability to hold body fluids and waste. I went home and discussed the issue with my children, Larry, and my bestie. With their help, I decided to go through with the procedure.

I had the first surgery in September 2011. My son brought me home and my bestie stayed by my bedside and took care of me. But the strong pain medication I was on made me think I had healed and could resume normal activities. Well, I was wrong. Healing would take longer for me, and I soon developed an anal ulcer. In March 2012, I had to undergo another operation. This made for two surgeries less than six months apart.

At this time, Larry was very concerned about me; he came and brought me home from the hospital after the second procedure and stayed to take care of me until all the medication from surgery had worn off. My son and bestie asked if I was okay with just Larry taking care of me, but I told them I was fine. Larry did a great job looking after me. I was his responsibility anyway. Plus, I needed to see whether he could function in a crisis.

God has shown me so much grace and mercy. I don't like wearing diapers, so I don't go far from home nowadays. Most of my trips are local. I no longer eat unhealthy foods often, either, so my health is easier for me to maintain. I am still trying to walk six miles again and have even designed another workout route that includes locations with restrooms to accommodate my disability. Regardless of the new challenges I face, there is no way I'm giving up. The key is for me to monitor my weight, no matter what.

Due to my lack of mobility, I gradually regained forty pounds. My doctor also recently diagnosed me with arthritis in both of my legs, which explains the extreme pain I have to endure every night. But I don't make any excuses for myself—I am still responsible for maintaining my weight loss. My spirit and heart receive constant nurture and encouragement from the Word of God, and drawing upon this, I have created new motivators to keep me focused. This book is just one way I hope to help others. In addition, I am in the process of creating a workout DVD for obese people who don't or can't really leave their homes; it will give me a chance to motivate them on a more personal level.

My granddaughter Shanice loves to run and play with me outside. I don't want my weight or other health issues to stop me from having fun with her. And I'd like to help others in my community, especially those facing health setbacks, find the strength and confidence to enjoy doing their favorite things, too. What a blessing God has given me to remain healthy enough to do so.

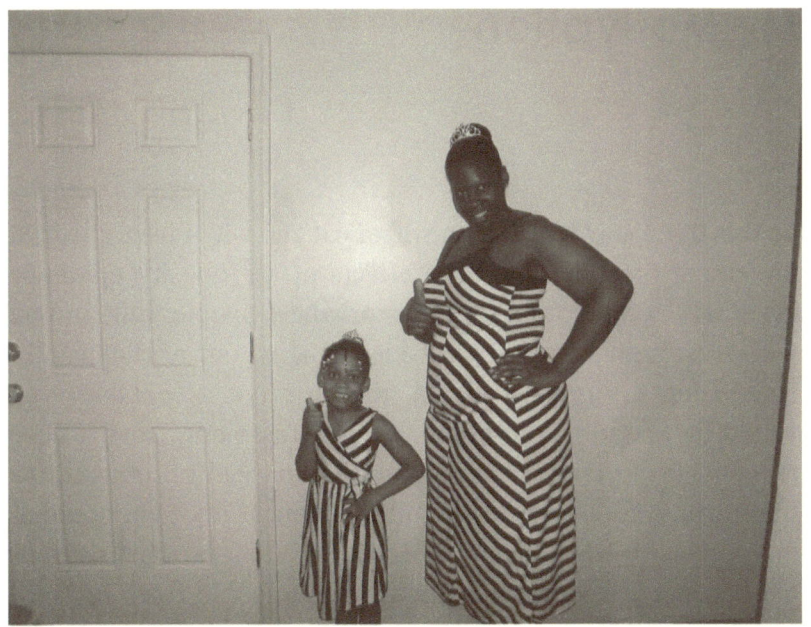

My Motivation

To this day, I stay focused on what I eat and why I have changed my eating lifestyle. I see the effects of the obesity epidemic every day. It has gotten to the point where people walk around with their stomachs and backsides hanging out of their clothing. When I was growing up, this was not acceptable—you would be teased to the point of embarrassment. Now, a huge percentage of people in this country face weight problems. It's the norm. Middle-aged men and women in my own community even use wheelchairs designed for seniors. This saddens me because I remember some of these people from my own childhood, back when they were fit and trim. The pressures of life have taken their toll on these brothers and sisters, and they seem to be handling this with food. But this just isn't the way to go. I know, because I've been there.

There is so much physical and emotional pain that comes along with taking this downward path. Being overweight is hard enough when you're young, but it only gets worse as you get older. Your muscles, tissues, and bones are not as strong anymore. The extra weight on your body feels like bricks causing pain beyond your imagination.

Often, the first places you feel the effects of your extra weight are in your legs and knees. My kneecap cartilage has been destroyed due to my obesity. And I can't just grow it back again! Once it's gone, it's gone. God gives each of us one body. It's a gift! So it's up to us to do everything we can to keep it healthy.

My personal goal is to lose thirty more pounds, just to make sure that I am at a comfortable weight for my age and physical strength level. But everyone's goals and needs will be different. One thing that really keeps me motivated, though, is being mindful of the health and weight problems of youths. Back in my day, there was no such thing as diagnosing children with high blood pressure and diabetes, and my heart aches now whenever I hear about it.

All my life, I suffered emotionally due to my weight and appearance. But I brought myself closer to God and now ask Him daily to help me push past my anxiety of crowds and others' judgment, and to help families in my community lose weight. There are many gyms and groups trying to help people trim down. But what if there's someone out there like me, who's ready to make changes but doesn't have a lot of money or suffers from a disability that doesn't allow them to go far from home? What if this person is shy and embarrassed?

Hopefully, this book and my DVD will allow me to reach all those in my community and communities like it who are seeking to achieve a healthier weight. I especially would like to get young adults thinking about their health and weight. If young adult parents start to become health conscience, then our future generations will have a much better chance of not having to battle diseases such as high blood pressure, diabetes, and high cholesterol. The cycle can be broken!

Losing weight is one of the rewards that comes with living a health-conscience lifestyle, but there are also many more. Being healthy allows you to take pleasure in even the most routine, everyday activities, such as going shopping, doing laundry, doing housework, and, yes, even parenting children. I notice that I don't easily become angry anymore, mainly because I use working out as a way to cope with my emotions.

Life comes with all sorts of obstacles, but when you're healthy, you can manage them more effectively. For example, no one wants to deal with cheating partners, including me. But nowadays, if I were to think my partner might be cheating, I wouldn't go through his phone or his pockets like I may have done in the past. I will exercise intensely, taking my frustration out on the fat in my body and mentally preparing for a possible breakup. Yes, you can prepare for situations like these the sensible way, instead of by eating a pint of ice cream and a whole cake!

My Outreach Efforts

It was very difficult for me to gain the courage to want to help other people with their weight issues. I had practiced hiding myself for over thirty years due to all the bullying and vicious name-calling I had endured for the majority of my life. Crowds and big events gave me anxiety. If I were to attend a party or some other type of celebration, I'd start shaking and sweating, and I'd lose all concentration. My use of language would become distorted and my sentences wouldn't make sense. I'd get the overwhelming feeling that everyone was talking, looking, and laughing at me, and those feelings would cause tremendous shame and embarrassment.

So I've had to work extremely hard to push past my fears to put myself out there and talk to others about weight loss, as well as the success I personally achieved without having much money. My baby sisters helped me start breaking through my anxiety by forcing me to attend family gatherings and events. I also started using my Facebook page to advertise my vision of weight loss for others. In addition, Larry began helping me use my body as a tool: he bought me my first spandex pants and waist-length blouse. The outfit attracted more attention to me—which caused me even more anxiety—but through God's grace, it also created a host of compliments from women, both young and old.

I was shocked to get compliments from my sisters. I was sure they would hate me or make me feel bad for now looking like a Coca-Cola bottle while there was still so much obesity in our community. A woman's body can distract even men who have good intentions. But my purpose would never be to use my body to hurt other sisters and their families or to damage their relationships. I want sisters to know that I am not influenced by the material things men can provide—I don't care about his money or about what he drives. What's important to me is how a man treats the woman he has at home. If a man can't respect his woman and be loyal to her, then he isn't worth the time. And with my previous relationship experience, I can spot a cheater from a mile away now.

My weight loss success has given me a new love for living life. I love taking pictures, making people laugh, and writing books and poetry. My friends and family won't stop clicking the camera. And the best part is, I don't mind anymore! I am complimented so much that I don't know what to do sometimes. But I don't ever let the attention go to my head. I don't use it as a reason to be mean to people. Instead, I stay focused and give glory to my Lord and Savior Jesus Christ for the body He blessed me with—the body that I now use to carry out His will.

The way I look at it, my body is a temple for Christ, and I try the best I can to take good care of it. No, I don't walk in perfection. But I am conscious of how I behave, how I carry myself, and the greater purpose I serve. It is now my aim to be a role model for girls and young women, especially the ones blessed with highly attractive bodies, because I want to help them understand just how special they are and teach them how to respect themselves and their bodies. Never in all my life would I have dreamed that God would one day give me such a beautiful figure. At forty-two, I am blessed to look ten years younger! And I have to admit, even though I have no desire to carry myself as a thirty-something-year-old woman, it sure feels good to look like one.

Whenever my granddaughter calls me grandma in public, it feels amazing—it shows me just how blessed and highly favored I am. I am a middle-aged grandma who is looking forward to her golden years. But sadly, I have not noticed many people from my generation in my community feeling good about themselves at this time in their lives. What I hear instead is them speaking of their anger and pain.

So I want to help. I've purchased a website for advertising and posting video clips. I have even reached out to local politicians and community officials for financial help in getting my weight loss message out. But so far, they've brushed me off and showed no interest in helping their communities. Reaching out to talk show hosts like Oprah, Dr. Drew, and Maury hasn't led anywhere yet, either. But I am not at all discouraged. I've just decided that I will put up my own money to help my community.

Symbolically speaking, my goal is to put tiaras on the head of every girl and young woman, especially those in their early teens through early twenties. I believe that if they are taught how to carry themselves as princesses, they will then treat their bodies the same way. It is God's grace that helps me press forward to help His children. People wonder why I care so much for others. The reason is this: the more I do for others, the more God does for me and my family. There are special blessings I seek straight from God, and no amount of money can buy them. What I pray for are continued peace, health, and sobriety. I would like for my children and family to always stay safe. I want my hubby, Lawrence, to keep that bright sparkle of love in his eyes for me for the rest of our lives. And, of course,

I wish to continue helping and encouraging others. Money simply can't buy these things!

PART III

The Creation of the Princess Plan

When I first devised the Princess Plan, I used myself as a model. I came up with a weight loss regimen specifically designed for me by me, and a treatment plan that would cater to my particular health needs and physical fitness. A princess is treated with respect and care; she is nurtured and protected at all times by her father or husband. So I said to myself, "That's it. People must care for themselves as a princess would, even if the person trying to lose weight is a man." All individuals must create special weight loss and maintenance routines for themselves—that is, regimens that are tailored to their bodies and cultural backgrounds.

The Princess Plan is a customized program. It's filled with suggestions, information, and tools designed to help participants create their own weight loss and maintenance regimens. Participants sit down, think about, and figure out the best foods to include in their routines. They find the safest exercises that are suitable for their bodies and strength levels, working out at a pace that is comfortable for them. When they're ready, they then learn how to gradually increase their workouts safely and effectively. Participants also learn skills for coping with their feelings, whether these emotions are good, bad, or indifferent. My personal philosophy is this: if a person takes the responsibility to design his or her own regimen, he or she is more likely to have long-term success.

Even though many people don't have a clear understanding of how they should treat their bodies, I try to explain it in terms that they can understand. One of my rules is that any food that does not have nutritional value should be considered garbage. For example, as a woman with a Southern background, I grew up loving soul food. But now I know that, under most circumstances, it's extremely unhealthy. Our African ancestors created dishes that would help them survive working long hours in the heat of the cotton fields during slavery. They had no other choice—they had to eat something or die. But over time, along with their recipes for soul food came genetic diseases like high blood pressure, diabetes, high cholesterol, and, of course, obesity. So the only way to prevent getting these diseases is to reverse the cycle by changing the way we eat.

I have followed many weight loss regimens that had no connection to my African American heritage. So until I created the Princess Plan, I couldn't fully understand why I couldn't lose weight. Fried chicken, macaroni and cheese, candied yams, collard greens, bacon and eggs with cheese grits, peach cobbler, cake, banana pudding, biscuits, cornbread, ham, pork chops, barbecue spareribs, steak and potatoes . . . They are delicious, but all these foods cause major problems for many people in the African American community. Why? Because no matter what the results or consequences of eating them are, they are very hard for many African Americans to resist.

How Does It Work and
Where Do You Start?

This is probably one of the first questions we ask ourselves when taking action to create change in our lives. With weight loss, the best place to start is in your mind. Your mindset about weight loss will determine your success. If you believe losing weight is too hard or that you are too overweight, then you won't be able to reach your goals. Maybe after trying every weight loss product that you could afford, joining all the local gyms, and having absolutely nothing work for you, you're sure there's nothing else you can do. Well, then guess what? The Princess Plan won't work for you, either! The reason is because your mindset has already determined the outcome.

The mind is the control center for every part of your body. There is a famous quote that says, "The mind is a terrible thing to waste." This is very true. Your mind determines your successes *and* failures, as well as your happiness, health, and hunger levels. Have you ever wondered why there are so many diet and exercise programs? Why do some work only for some people and not for everyone who purchases them? The truth is that all these programs have the potential to work. But because our mindsets are different at certain times in our lives, whether or not these programs will work for you will depend on whether or not you are ready to make them work for you. So when trying to lose weight, you must have a strong mindset at all times—before, during, and after. If you don't, you risk not only not being able to shed pounds but also unconsciously gaining them back, depending on what is happening in your life. Your mindset is what monitors your weight loss and your success maintaining it.

Once I understood this important concept, I was able to succeed. I had tried Weight Watchers, Lucille Roberts, Curves, Total Gym, Body by Jake, Slim-Fast, Six-Week Body Makeover—none of these programs worked for me! What finally did work, though, was coming up with my own personalized weight loss regimen. I created my own eating habits, I created my own workout routine, and I created my own frequency of working out. It's *my* weight loss regimen. I have gotten good information and ideas from many weight loss programs, including the ones I tried in the past, but I didn't own them—I didn't make them *mine*. So I'm confident that once you find exactly what works for you, you'll be successful, too. That's what my Princess Plan is designed to help you do.

One of the biggest mistakes successful weight loss participates make is forgetting that reckless eating was the cause of their weight gain. Their mindset somehow starts to justify that eating recklessly again is okay after they've had long periods of weight loss success. These people aren't aware that weight maintenance success is supported by a health-conscious-eating mindset. It's also important to remember that, if you're trying to lose weight, you must not give up on yourself. When I regained weight during the course of my rehabilitation after having surgery, I immediately sought help from my doctors—I didn't just give up! Right now, my health condition is not the same as when I first started my weight loss routine. But what happened to my body was beyond my control. So I accepted that. And I started working on a way to continue losing weight and stay healthy that will accommodate my current health status. I lost 130 pounds but gained back forty. But I am very aware that if I don't do anything to get back on track, the other ninety pounds will find me sooner or later! And I'm not about to let that happen! The key is to always remain conscious of your goals and make whatever changes necessary to staying on track.

You Need God or a Higher Power

I know there are some people who dislike the idea of telling their troubles to God or a higher power whom they don't believe in or ever had a relationship with. The lack of knowledge in this area saddens me. My personal experience and suggestions are all I can share. It is not my goal to preach or convert you to a specific belief system. I'd just like to express how grateful I am not to have to go through life without my Lord and Savior Jesus Christ and the strength I have found in Him. During every struggle I had, especially those with my substance abuse and HIV status, I went to Him. So many of my community members could not do anything for me except express pity, shame, and blame. And although I am thankful for my family and true friends' support, I know I would not be where I am today without God's divine guidance and love.

Now more than ever, there seems to be a need for God's help in order to cope with our lives and all the stressful and painful situations that arise. The strength it takes to emotionally survive broken relationships, health conditions, death, single parenting, unemployment, and homelessness is far more than what we can provide ourselves on our own. At this point, a huge majority of our country has been classified as overweight or obese. Food seems to have become a major way of emotionally dealing with these situations. There was a time when we could rely and call on our pastors, leaders, and elders. They would pray for us and support us until we conquered our hardships. But this is not as much the case today. Too many of our leaders are more interested now in fame and money. And our elders are being weakened by disease.

So it's extremely important for us to take extra responsibility for ourselves and remember what we learned while growing up in God-loving households. Many of us were taught to be baptized and to go directly to God when things got tough. I firmly believe that God is graceful and merciful, and that He will always love all His children, no matter what. All we need is a little faith, and God will take care of the rest. He does what His Word promises—all we have to do is ask to receive the wisdom and knowledge of His teachings.

I know some of us have been frightened into submission by being taught to fear God and His authority. This has unfortunately caused a lot of rebellion against Him. But God is forgiving, and it is never too late for anyone, regardless of your mistakes in life, to create a new relationship with Him. For me, I personally can't imagine a world without God.

If you are on a mission to lose weight, I truly believe in my heart that God will help you accomplish your goals if you have faith in Him. Despite every obstacle I met throughout my life—being bullied, doing drugs, drinking alcohol, prostituting, being diagnosed with HIV, smoking cigarettes, dealing with cheating partners, being separated from my children, gaining weight, suffering from arthritis, having to undergo surgery, and so much more—God never forsook me. So after all I've been through and survived, I can't express enough the importance of tapping into God's power throughout your own weight loss process.

Weight loss and weight maintenance are not easy, especially with the many unhealthy fast food restaurants that have overtaken our low-income communities. Temptation does not discriminate; it is capable of harming whoever crosses its path, regardless of their background. That's why I am convinced that a connection to God is greatly needed to fight this risk. So as someone who has a wonderful relationship with my Lord and Savior Jesus Christ, I strongly suggest that you get with either Him or a higher power of your choice.

Motivators and Consistency

Motivators are anyone and anything that make you feel good and help you stay on track. Family and friends can be motivators. A motivator can also be any situation that pushes you forward—believe it or not, even stressful situations such as divorces or deaths can be motivators. Compliments from attractive people—especially those you may have a crush on—are motivators. The way *you* see yourself in the mirror can be a motivator. Old pictures of you can be motivators. New clothes that fit your new figure can be motivators, too. Whatever helps to keep you focused on your weight loss goals is a motivator. And the more motivators you have, the better off you are. Of course, every individual's motivators will differ, but this is okay. So don't freak out or judge and undermine yourself if what motivates you is not the same as what motivates someone else. Your motivators are tailored to suit *you*!

Consistency is a very important concept to understand, too; your weight loss and weight maintenance depend on it. Once you've set a goal, you have to stick to it. Maybe you want to be part of the crew who has decided to lose weight. The intention is there, but deep down, you may not be totally ready because you still want to eat junk and fast foods. Let me tell you, if you truly feel like this, then you're going to be pushing a boulder up a mountain. You may get started with a soup-and-salad diet or a liquid diet. But in no time at all, you'll feel like you're starving. It will become easy for you to justify your decision to break your healthy diet and start binging. Before you know it, you'll be gaining even more weight, and by the time you finally come to your senses, extreme damage will have been done. The disappointment will lead to feelings of defeat and even more overeating as the vicious cycle begins all over again. You can't practice healthy living on Monday and switch to reckless eating on Tuesday! So if you're not totally ready for a lifestyle change, don't start until you are—it will only cause you more harm than good!

PART IV

How Did We Gain Weight?

I am sure many of you are kicking yourself wondering how you gained so much weight. Maybe you were lean and trim at one time in your life and would never have imagined yourself gaining as much weight as you have. I totally understand your concern, even though I actually have been overweight for most of my life.

As I explored the many reasons for my own weight gain, I realized that not only did I have very poor eating habits, but that I was also too ashamed of my obese appearance to exercise. The worst part was that I mentally accepted myself this way and concluded that I had no choice but to stay obese until I die. This acceptance eventually really began to bother me, though, because at six feet tall and four hundred pounds, I was not ideal wife and mother material.

My research also led me to find out that all sorts of things can cause weight gain, such as stress, unbalanced thyroid function, medications, sickness, and mental health issues. So at one point, I realized that, no matter what the reason is for gaining weight, there has to be a *solution*.

One solution is to start or reboot your metabolism. Your metabolism is like a machine your body uses to burn fat. Well, what gets your metabolism going? Exercise. I consider exercise to be any kind of consistent movement that causes you to exert energy and sweat. Even homemaker chores and babysitting can be good workouts; if you get tired while doing this kind of activity, then it is a workout.

Another question to ask yourself is, "Why do I want to lose weight?" You need to be very careful in examining your reasons. I sponsor over one hundred weight loss participants and have found that every one of them has a different reason for wanting to lose weight. Some have said they need to, many have said they have to, others have said it's healthier, a few have said their families and doctors suggested it, and several have said they want to relieve the physical pain caused by their extra weight. But not one person has said, "I want to lose weight because *I* want to." This is often the most powerful reason of all.

Your personal reason for losing weight will be your regular tool and your constant reminder. How you will maintain your weight loss is also something you'll have to consider. If you start on a weight loss program only because someone else recommended it, even though this might be cool to start, you likely will not be able to maintain it. You must accept and commit to this process on your own accord and personalize it to be able to enjoy long-term success. This is why I believe that creating your own weight loss regimen is so effective. *You* create and apply it to *yourself*.

Think of it this way: Even celebrities and wealthy people have sometimes failed to achieve their weight loss goals. They probably have producers and managers talking at them all day about weight loss, so these people lose weight under obligation. But as soon as their managers' and producers' backs are turned and the spotlights go out, the eating binges begin. The pressure of having to lose weight for the wrong reasons becomes very stressful for anyone of any social class. That's why it's so

Latonya R. Baskerville

important to be true and good to yourself first. If you're moti-
vating yourself with the right reasons, you can make anything
happen!

Creating Your Exercise Regimen

Creating your own exercise regimen simply means finding comfortable exercises that work for you. Not all people can move the same way. For example, I don't jog, but my father was a jogger for over twenty-five years. It worked for him, but the results of jogging for some people can be damage to the ankles and knees. So I decided jogging wouldn't be for me. My dad told me that walking would be a great workout, though, and that I could do it for as long as I live without worrying about damaging anything in my legs. So I took it up as my personal, preferred way to exercise.

When I first started walking, it was painful because my muscles were not used to it. Once my body adjusted, however, I started power-twist-walking, a technique I learned from a cousin. You need to give your body time to adjust. This is key, because if you don't keep this in mind, you can get discouraged very quickly. I also especially want to encourage you not to become disappointed by exercise videos. They teach many techniques, but you might not be able to keep up with the actors in them because those people have been working out for years. This is why you have to find what works for you. There are some who love bike riding. Many people enjoy going to gyms and aerobics classes. Others like dancing. It doesn't matter how you choose to exercise as long as you sweat!

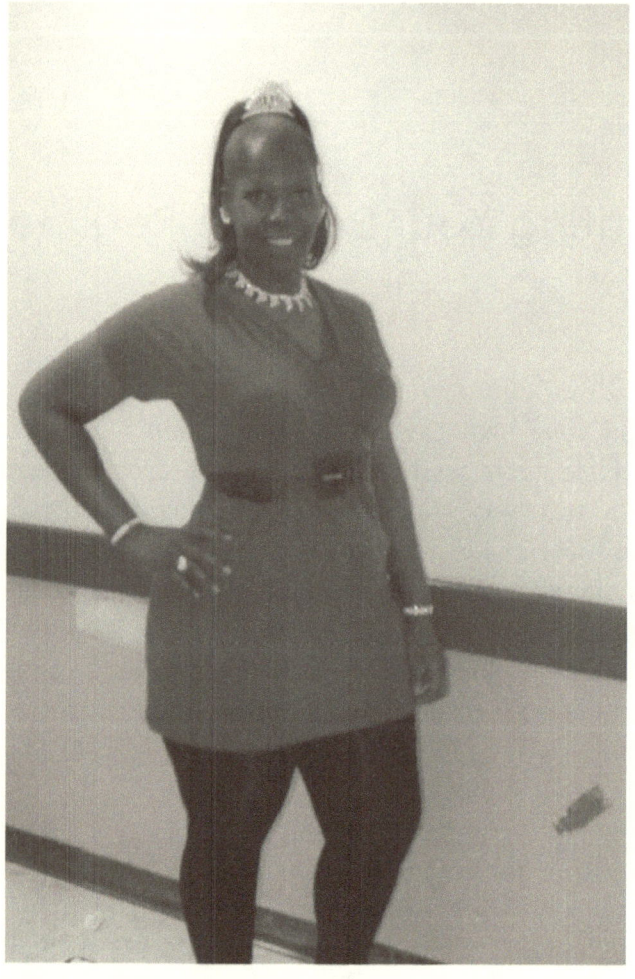

Again, it's important to remember that the exercise regimen you create is something that you do for your own health and well-being. The commitment to work out is in your hands! I can't emphasize it enough: this is a *lifestyle commitment* that should last you for the rest of your life. Too many people seem to believe that they can work out until the weight comes off and then stop. It makes me so sad when I see people's weight go up and down because they've failed to commit. It is extremely frustrating when you achieve your weight goal but gain it right back within a few months. And this is exactly what makes people decide to give up and convince themselves that they must accept that they will remain overweight or obese for the rest of their lives. Those are thoughts of defeat. I've had them and I know where they come from: Satan. He really does want you to live in pain, misery, and defeat in every area of your life. But you cannot let him win! The reality is, things *are* going to happen in our lives that are out of our control. So instead of letting these situations bring us down, we must prepare to meet our challenges, accept what we can't change, keep the faith, and do the best we can under our circumstances.

Creating Your Favorite
Low-Calorie Diet

Creating my favorite low-calorie diet was a lot of fun for me. The best part was that I could still enjoy delicious foods while eating healthily. For example, I dropped pork and beef and substituted them with chicken and turkey. Instead of eating white rice, white bread, and potatoes, I now eat more whole grains, which can taste just as good—and, of course, they're better for you! I don't drink whole milk, but I love fat-free milk and soy milk. Sodas and sugary fruit juices are no longer a part of my diet; water is now my drink of choice. In fact, I recently learned a great way to make "soda" using seltzer water and flavor drops.

Making similar kinds of adjustments to your eating habits will play a major part in your weight loss process. Don't worry, you won't have to give up eating the foods you love. But you will have to modify them so that they're healthier and have less calories. Fruits can replace sugary fruit-flavored candies and fruit juices. Crunchy roasted nuts can be substituted for greasy potato chips. Frozen yogurt can step in for full-fat ice cream.

Cooking healthier won't be as hard as you might think, either. I used to watch one of my cousins prepare dishes, and I'd notice that he always removed the skin from the chicken.

He would also never fry food—he'd even boil ground beef to make burgers. At first, I thought he had lost his mind. What he was doing seemed funny to me. But I still paid attention and asked questions, and looking back now, I am so grateful that he allowed me to learn from him. Just because something is done differently doesn't mean it's going to turn out badly!

There is no such thing as a "magic low-calorie diet" that will fit everyone. And it might take a little time to find what works best for you. As you begin to create your personalized meal plans, though, you'll find all sorts of foods that are much better for you than what you might be used to eating now. Yes, it will take patience and commitment. But again, making a commitment to eat healthier is also making a commitment to live a *longer* and *happier* life.

Dealing with Your Emotions and Maintaining Your Weight

Many people may think that emotions don't play a part in their weight management. The fact is, though, that they really do. Every time I used to overeat, it was linked to how I was feeling. Whether I was happy, sad, angry, mourning, nervous, embarrassed, scared, frustrated, or anxious, I dealt with my emotions by eating food. It is so important to learn to deal with your feelings in a more productive way.

The older you become, the harder it gets to shed excess weight. In addition, the longer you let yourself live unhealthily, the more danger you face of developing serious weight-related health issues. I am extremely grateful to God for giving me the energy and willpower to start my weight loss process when I did because I simply don't have the same stamina anymore. At this point in my life, I am somewhat confined to my home and don't have the financial resources to create a home gym for myself, though I have designed an exercise plan that works around my current situation. We never know what tomorrow will bring. But we do have today. So if you've been thinking about losing weight, I encourage you to get started sooner than later!

Again, you have to take hold of your emotions. You must first learn to think positively, and then use this to continue driving you toward your goals. No matter whether I feel good, bad, or indifferent, I work out. I may not feel like it at first, but once I get going, my mind is freed of all negativity and worries. My workouts are outside, so I am watched from the time I leave my home until the time I return. It makes me self-conscious sometimes, but I don't let my broken-down self-esteem dictate my desire to exercise—I stay focused and I remain in control of my success. *I do me!*

I want to teach you to do the same thing. I personally have experienced what it feels like to lose loved ones through death, separation, cheating, and changes of heart. But I also know now that hurting myself with food definitely won't bring them back. I had to learn a lot of lessons the hard way, including the fact that money can't buy love or acceptance. You've got to love yourself first. The rest will follow.

Life is given when you're born and all sorts of feelings are experienced every step of the way. There are never any guarantees. That's just the way things go. So you must learn how to identify your feelings, accept them, and then go through them. Family, true friends, and even medical professionals can help you; you shouldn't ever have to feel like you're all alone. And if you remain positive and keep the faith, despite life's trials and tribulations, you will find that you can find a solution, survive, and succeed.

Thank you so much for purchasing and reading my book. May the God of your understanding bless you with a long life and prosperity. In the name of my Lord and Savior Jesus Christ, amen.

Though your contributions and donations Training Individuals Make Better Attitudes Inc A section 501c3 not for profit organization, We can continue to educate, encourage and Inspire families in the community and all around the world.

We train individuals in areas of stress and struggle. We believe if a family is trained in the areas In which they struggle, then that family can resolve their own issues.

If you want to support us please email us at: trainingindividuals2014@gmail.com

PART V
POEMS

Whose Kids Are These?

This is a special poem dedicated to all the families who lost loved ones to senseless crimes committed by other people's kids.

Whose kids are these?These are the babies born addicted, left on steps,
With nobody to feed them, babies born to abuse and neglect,
Some parents in recovery and some who forget.

These are the kids who suffered despair,
Crying all night but no one cared.
Adopted by families with no physical match,
Dumped at fourteen, then they mentally snapped.

These are the kids who grew up to hate,
Thinking their life was a big mistake.
When they have children, they will teach them the same,
That taking a life is a daily game.

They have no fear, they don't know God,
And their parents just taught them that life is hard.
They steal when they can, to kill is a must,
Fuck this world, there's no one they trust.

Please stop the violence, children.
I know life seems hard,
But Jesus is here and He knows God.

He gave his life for you and for me,
Just look in the Bible, Isaiah 53.[29]

I am living proof that all can change,
And proud to announce God knows my name.
He wrote it in heaven,
Just check the Bible, John 15:1–27.[30]

Where Is the Village?

Who knows where's the village that raised blessed kids,
That respected adults and passed down baby cribs?

Who knows where's the village that knew all families by name,
That taught children well and spared them of shame?

Who knows where's the village where children called you
Mister or Miss?
I can't remember the last time I heard a child say this.

Who knows where's the village where children go to bed?
Now they're missing for weeks, and some are found dead.

Who knows where's the village that had teachers who cared?
Now they're sexing and molesting them
and beating them with chairs.

Who knows where's the village where we all wanted to live,
Where black stuck together and loved each other's kids?

Who knows where's the village where guns were colored and
used for fun?
The biggest one held the most water, and if you
got hit you were drenched and stunned.

Well, I guess there's no village or black communities that are
strong,
So they murder our children all night long.

Can You Help?

Can *you* help rear a bruised and battered kid,
Teaching them morals and values like our forefathers did?

Can *you* help even if they're grown
And have many children of their own?

Can *you* help give them nurture, show care,
Provide added security to reclaim their life without any fear?

Can *you* help teach them the definition of hope
And the importance of using their right to vote?

Can *you* help them gain and build self-esteem
So they will stop killing each other all in the name of da green?

Can *you* help show them how civil people behave
So cops won't have reasons to put them in graves?

Can *you* help show them that an education is an investment in self,
That skills, not drugs, build financial wealth?

Can *you* help show that the world does give a fuck,
And that employers will hire if they pull their pants up?

Can *you* help make them understand:
What you put in your life is what you get out,
It has nothing to do with the white man.

Not Your Problem

You think it's not your problem the way the children behave,
They're fighting and killing each other, going to early graves,
Sleeping at Port Authority and eating straight off the ground,
Breaking into a house, cutting up a family,
and no body parts are found.

You think it's not your problem because your children are safe,
Until your thirteen-year-old runs home and tells you he was
raped.
Now his mind is distorted, and he thinks the world is a bluff,
He can't cope with life, so he starts smoking stuff.
He is all messed up, and you can't help him out,
You start to wish you wouldn't have let him out the house.

You think it's not your problem because you live in the hills,
Little do you know they travel there often, seeking new thrills.
They could care less about your Cosby sweater and huskabull
home,
About you praying and laying for your wife and daughters to
be left alone.
No matter how much money you have or what you saved,
A racist knows his kind, and you will always be a slave.
They will never let you close or near their homes,
So do yourself a favor and take care of your own.

Don't Let It Hit Home

Don't let it hit home,
Help a troubled person feel loved when they feel alone.
We all need nurture, especially when we're grown,
It's not always about money, you could pick up a phone.
It doesn't cost anything to say, "How do you do?"
Listen for a while, let them vent, then say, "Don't worry, I love you."
To make it here, we can't use rifles,
We need loving people, even Jesus had twelve disciples.
They followed him around with love and loyalty, there was nothing greater,
Of course, God knew which one would deny Him and who was the trader.
We still need each other, even those who lie,
And it's gonna be that way until the day we die.
Empowering other people is the glory of my life,
I lived through horrible situations, especially pain and strife.
Now putting me aside strengthens my own growth,
I wouldn't trade it for the world, not everyone cuts your throat.

Christian Life

How do you measure my Christian life?
Is it determined by my pain and strife?
Is it measured through my goods and worth?
Or is it measured by the way I curse?
Is it measured by my life knocks and—oops—
My past as a prostitute?
Is it measured by my lies or truths?
Or is it measured only by you?
My relationship to Christ is approved by whom?
He gave His life for me and for you.
The children of God need to win more souls
And stop attacking each other with judgmental woes.
We will all get a chance at the end of our fight
To show our Savior what we did in this life.

Do You See Your Part?

When you look at the world, where do you see your part?
Can you see the lost souls with broken hearts?
Or do you see money, sex, and lots of bling?
Are you working mostly for material things?
If so, that's fine, you can have it your way,
But when do you stop, because styles change every day?
When I needed more meaning, I looked at me no more,
I started seeing lost souls, so my knees hit the floor.
I asked my Lord, "Father, can I help?"
He answered, "My child, your path is dealt.
Just walk hard in faith and not by sight,
I'll show you the right people, you will see the light.
Don't feed no evil or do things out of spite,
Because vengeance is mine, and it's not your fight."

My Body Belongs to Christ

My body belongs to Christ,
And I know my butt is big and y'all call it nice.
My body belongs to Christ,
Because He was beaten for my sins until He gave up His life.
My body belongs to Christ,
That which is done on earth shall be done in the afterlife.
My body belongs to Christ,
Now that you know, I want to please Him and give Him
delight.
My body belongs to Christ,
Because He guided me from the depths of hell back into the
light.
My body belongs to Christ,
Which means I don't abuse it or get into unnecessary fights.
My body belongs to Christ,
I won't use it to destroy relationships and families in the
middle of the night.
My body belongs to Christ,
If you don't understand what I just said, I will gladly say it
twice.
My body belongs to Christ,
If you agree with what I'm saying, you shouldn't
have any problems giving Him your life.

(Endnotes)

1. A wife of noble character who can find? She is worth far more than rubies. Her husband has full confidence in her and lacks nothing of value. She brings him good, not harm, all the days of her life. She selects wool and flax and works with eager hands. She is like the merchant ships, bringing her food from afar. She gets up while it is still night; she provides food for her family and portions for her female servants. She considers a field and buys it; out of her earnings she plants a vineyard. She sets about her work vigorously; her arms are strong for her tasks. She sees that her trading is profitable, and her lamp does not go out at night. In her hand she holds the distaff and grasps the spindle with her fingers. She opens her arms to the poor and extends her hands to the needy. When it snows, she has no fear for her household; for all of them are clothed in scarlet. She makes coverings for her bed; she is clothed in fine linen and purple. Her husband is respected at the city gate, where he takes his seat among the elders of the land. She makes linen garments and sells them, and supplies the merchants with sashes. She

is clothed with strength and dignity; she can laugh at the days to come. She speaks with wisdom, and faithful instruction is on her tongue. She watches over the affairs of her household and does not eat the bread of idleness. Her children arise and call her blessed; her husband also, and he praises her: "Many women do noble things, but you surpass them all." Charm is deceptive, and beauty is fleeting; but a woman who fears the LORD is to be praised. Honor her for all that her hands have done, and let her works bring her praise at the city gate. (Proverbs 31:10–31)

2. In him we were also chosen, having been predestined according to the plan of him who works out everything in conformity with the purpose of his will. (Ephesians 1:11)

3. Do not judge, and you will not be judged. Do not condemn, and you will not be condemned. Forgive, and you will be forgiven. Give, and it will be given to you. A good measure, pressed down, shaken together and running over, will be poured into your lap. For with the measure you use, it will be measured to you. (Luke 6:37–38)

So in everything, do to others what you would have them do to you, for this sums up the Law and the Prophets. (Matthew 7:12)

4. Why do you look at the speck of sawdust in your brother's eye and pay no attention to the plank in your own eye? How can you say to your brother, "Let me take the speck out of your eye," when all the time there is a plank in your own eye? You hypocrite, first take the plank out

of your own eye, and then you will see clearly to remove the speck from your brother's eye. (Matthew 7:3–5)

5. Do your best to present yourself to God as one approved, a worker who does not need to be ashamed and who correctly handles the word of truth. (2 Timothy 2:15)

6. Concerning the prophets: My heart is broken within me; all my bones tremble. I am like a drunken man, like a strong man overcome by wine, because of the LORD and his holy words. The land is full of adulterers; because of the curse the land lies parched and the pastures in the wilderness are withered. The prophets follow an evil course and use their power unjustly. "Both prophet and priest are godless; even in my temple I find their wickedness," declares the LORD. "Therefore their path will become slippery; they will be banished to darkness and there they will fall. I will bring disaster on them in the year they are punished," declares the LORD. "Among the prophets of Samaria I saw this repulsive thing: They prophesied by Baal and led my people Israel astray. And among the prophets of Jerusalem I have seen something horrible: They commit adultery and live a lie. They strengthen the hands of evildoers, so that not one of them turns from their wickedness. They are all like Sodom to me; the people of Jerusalem are like Gomorrah." Therefore this is what the LORD Almighty says concerning the prophets: "I will make them eat bitter food and drink poisoned water, because from the prophets of Jerusalem ungodliness has spread throughout the land." This is what the LORD Almighty says: "Do not listen to what the prophets are prophesying to you; they fill you with false hopes. They speak visions from their own minds, not from the

mouth of the LORD. They keep saying to those who despise me, 'The LORD says: You will have peace.' And to all who follow the stubbornness of their hearts they say, 'No harm will come to you.' But which of them has stood in the council of the LORD to see or to hear his word? Who has listened and heard his word? See, the storm of the LORD will burst out in wrath, a whirlwind swirling down on the heads of the wicked. The anger of the LORD will not turn back until he fully accomplishes the purposes of his heart. In days to come you will understand it clearly. I did not send these prophets, yet they have run with their message; I did not speak to them, yet they have prophesied. But if they had stood in my council, they would have proclaimed my words to my people and would have turned them from their evil ways and from their evil deeds. "Am I only a God nearby," declares the LORD, "and not a God far away?" "Who can hide in secret places so that I cannot see them?" declares the LORD. "Do not I fill heaven and earth?" declares the LORD. "I have heard what the prophets say who prophesy lies in my name. They say, 'I had a dream! I had a dream!' How long will this continue in the hearts of these lying prophets, who prophesy the delusions of their own minds? They think the dreams they tell one another will make my people forget my name, just as their ancestors forgot my name through Baal worship. Let the prophet who has a dream recount the dream, but let the one who has my word speak it faithfully. For what has straw to do with grain?" declares the LORD. "Is not my word like fire," declares the LORD, "and like a hammer that breaks a rock in pieces?" "Therefore," declares the LORD, "I am against the prophets who steal from one another words supposedly from me. Yes," declares the LORD, "I am against the prophets who wag their own tongues and yet declare, 'The LORD declares.' Indeed, I am against those who prophesy false dreams," declares the LORD. "They tell them and lead my people astray with their reckless lies, yet I did not send or appoint them. They do not benefit these people in the least," declares the LORD. "When these people, or a prophet or a priest, ask you, 'What is the message from the LORD?' say to them, 'What message? I will forsake you, declares the LORD.' If a prophet or a priest or anyone else claims, 'This is a message from the LORD,' I will punish them and their household. This is what each of you keeps saying to your friends and other Israelites: 'What is the LORD's answer?' or 'What has the LORD spoken?' But you must not mention 'a message from the LORD' again, because each one's word becomes their own message. So you distort the words of the living God, the LORD Almighty, our God. This is what you keep saying to a prophet: 'What is the LORD's answer to you?' or 'What has the LORD spoken?' Although you claim, 'This is a message from the LORD,' this is what the LORD says: You used the words, 'This is a message from the LORD,' even though I told you that you must not claim, 'This is a message from the LORD.' Therefore, I will surely forget you and cast you out of my presence along with the city I gave to you and your ancestors. I will bring on you everlasting disgrace—everlasting shame that will not be forgotten." (Jeremiah 23:9–40)

7. Come, all you who are thirsty, come to the waters; and you who have no money, come, buy and eat! Come, buy wine and milk without money and without cost. Why spend money on what is not bread, and your labor on what does not satisfy? Listen, listen to me, and eat what is good, and you will delight in the richest of fare. Give ear and come to me; listen, that you may live. I will make an

everlasting covenant with you, my faithful love promised to David. See, I have made him a witness to the peoples, a ruler and commander of the peoples. Surely you will summon nations you know not, and nations you do not know will come running to you, because of the LORD your God, the Holy One of Israel, for he has endowed you with splendor. Seek the LORD while he may be found; call on him while he is near. Let the wicked forsake their ways and the unrighteous their thoughts. Let them turn to the LORD, and he will have mercy on them, and to our God, for he will freely pardon. "For my thoughts are not your thoughts, neither are your ways my ways," declares the LORD. "As the heavens are higher than the earth, so are my ways higher than your ways and my thoughts than your thoughts. (Isaiah 55:1–9)

8. I am the LORD, and there is no other; apart from me there is no God. I will strengthen you, though you have not acknowledged me, so that from the rising of the sun to the place of its setting people may know there is none besides me. I am the LORD, and there is no other. I form the light and create darkness, I bring prosperity and create disaster; I, the LORD, do all these things. (Isaiah 45:5–7)

For this is what the LORD says—he who created the heavens, he is God; he who fashioned and made the earth, he founded it; he did not create it to be empty, but formed it to be inhabited—he says: "I am the LORD, and there is no other. I have not spoken in secret, from somewhere in a land of darkness; I have not said to Jacob's descendants, 'Seek me in vain.' I, the LORD, speak the truth; I declare what is right. Gather together and come; assemble, you fugitives from the nations. Ignorant are those who carry about idols of wood, who pray to gods that cannot save. Declare what is to be, present it—let them take counsel together. Who foretold this long ago, who declared it from the distant past? Was it not I, the LORD? And there is no God apart from me, a righteous God and a Savior; there is none but me. Turn to me and be saved, all you ends of the earth; for I am God, and there is no other. By myself I have sworn, my mouth has uttered in all integrity a word that will not be revoked: Before me every knee will bow; by me every tongue will swear. They will say of me, 'In the LORD alone are deliverance and strength.'" All who have raged against him will come to him and be put to shame. But all the descendants of Israel will find deliverance in the LORD and will make their boast in him. (Isaiah 45:18–25)

Even to your old age and gray hairs I am he, I am he who will sustain you. I have made you and I will carry you; I will sustain you and I will rescue you. With whom will you compare me or count me equal? To whom will you liken me that we may be compared? (Isaiah 46:4–5)

Remember the former things, those of long ago; I am God, and there is no other; I am God, and there is none like me. I make known the end from the beginning, from ancient times, what is still to come. I say, "My purpose will stand, and I will do all that I please." (Isaiah 46:9–10)

9. I keep asking that the God of our Lord Jesus Christ, the glorious Father, may give you the Spirit of wisdom and revelation, so that you may know him better. I pray that the eyes of your heart may be enlightened in order that you may know the hope to which he has called you, the riches of his glorious inheritance in his holy people, and

his incomparably great power for us who believe. That power is the same as the mighty strength. (Ephesians 1:17–19)

10. Your word is a lamp for my feet, a light on my path. I have taken an oath and confirmed it, that I will follow your righteous laws. I have suffered much; preserve my life, LORD, according to your word. Accept, LORD, the willing praise of my mouth, and teach me your laws. Though I constantly take my life in my hands, I will not forget your law. The wicked have set a snare for me, but I have not strayed from your precepts. Your statutes are my heritage forever; they are the joy of my heart. My heart is set on keeping your decrees to the very end. (Psalm 119:105–112)

11. My son, pay attention to what I say; turn your ear to my words. Do not let them out of your sight, keep them within your heart; for they are life to those who find them and health to one's whole body. (Proverbs 4:20–22)

12. He replied, "Because you have so little faith. Truly I tell you, if you have faith as small as a mustard seed, you can say to this mountain, 'Move from here to there,' and it will move. Nothing will be impossible for you." (Matthew 17:20)

13. For God so loved the world that he gave his one and only Son, that whoever believes in him shall not perish but have eternal life. (John 3:16)

14. "Have faith in God," Jesus answered. "Truly I tell you, if anyone says to this mountain, 'Go, throw yourself into

the sea,' and does not doubt in their heart but believes that what they say will happen, it will be done for them." (Mark 11:22–23)

15. For I am convinced that neither death nor life, neither angels nor demons, neither the present nor the future, nor any powers, neither height nor depth, nor anything else in all creation, will be able to separate us from the love of God that is in Christ Jesus our Lord. (Romans 8:38–39)

Give thanks to the LORD, for he is good; his love endures forever. Let the redeemed of the LORD tell their story— those he redeemed from the hand of the foe, those he gathered from the lands, from east and west, from north and south. Some wandered in desert wastelands, finding no way to a city where they could settle. They were hungry and thirsty, and their lives ebbed away. Then they cried out to the LORD in their trouble, and he delivered them from their distress. He led them by a straight way to a city where they could settle. Let them give thanks to the LORD for his unfailing love and his wonderful deeds for mankind, for he satisfies the thirsty and fills the hungry with good things. Some sat in darkness, in utter darkness, prisoners suffering in iron chains, because they rebelled against God's commands and despised the plans of the Most High. So he subjected them to bitter labor; they stumbled, and there was no one to help. Then they cried to the LORD in their trouble, and he saved them from their distress. He brought them out of darkness, the utter darkness, and broke away their chains. Let them give thanks to the LORD for his unfailing love and his wonderful deeds for mankind, for he breaks down gates of bronze and cuts through bars of iron. Some became fools through their rebellious ways and suffered affliction because of their iniquities. They loathed all food and drew near the gates of death. Then they cried to the LORD in their trouble, and he saved them from their distress. He sent out his word and healed them; he rescued them from the grave. Let them give thanks to the LORD for his unfailing love and his wonderful deeds for mankind. Let them sacrifice thank offerings and tell of his works with songs of joy. Some went out on the sea in ships; they were merchants on the mighty waters. They saw the works of the LORD, his wonderful deeds in the deep. For he spoke and stirred up a tempest that lifted high the waves. They mounted up to the heavens and went down to the depths; in their peril their courage melted away. They reeled and staggered like drunkards; they were at their wits' end. Then they cried out to the LORD in their trouble, and he brought them out of their distress. He stilled the storm to a whisper; the waves of the sea were hushed. They were glad when it grew calm, and he guided them to their desired haven. Let them give thanks to the LORD for his unfailing love and his wonderful deeds for mankind. Let them exalt him in the assembly of the people and praise him in the council of the elders. He turned rivers into a desert, flowing springs into thirsty ground, and fruitful land into a salt waste, because of the wickedness of those who lived there. He turned the desert into pools of water and the parched ground into flowing springs; there he brought the hungry to live, and they founded a city where they could settle. They sowed fields and planted vine-yards that yielded a fruitful harvest; he blessed them, and their numbers greatly increased, and he did not let their herds diminish. Then their numbers decreased, and they were humbled by oppression, calamity and sorrow; he who pours contempt on nobles made them wander in a

trackless waste. But he lifted the needy out of their affliction and increased their families like flocks. The upright
see and rejoice, but all the wicked shut their mouths. Let
the one who is wise heed these things and ponder the
loving deeds of the LORD. (Psalm 107)

Declare what is to be, present it—let them take counsel
together. Who foretold this long ago, who declared it
from the distant past? Was it not I, the LORD? And there
is no God apart from me, a righteous God and a Savior;
there is none but me. Turn to me and be saved, all you
ends of the earth; for I am God, and there is no other. By
myself I have sworn, my mouth has uttered in all integrity
a word that will not be revoked: Before me every knee
will bow; by me every tongue will swear. They will say
of me, "In the LORD alone are deliverance and strength."
All who have raged against him will come to him and be
put to shame. But all the descendants of Israel will find
deliverance in the LORD and will make their boast in
him. (Isaiah 45:21–25)

16. Please see note 1.

17. Jesus went throughout Galilee, teaching in their synagogues, proclaiming the good news of the kingdom, and
healing every disease and sickness among the people.
News about him spread all over Syria, and people brought
to him all who were ill with various diseases, those suffering severe pain, the demon-possessed, those having sei-
zures, and the paralyzed; and he healed them. (Matthew
4:23–24)

18. But he was pierced for our transgressions, he was
crushed for our iniquities; the punishment that brought

us peace was on him, and by his wounds we are healed. We all, like sheep, have gone astray, each of us has turned to our own way; and the LORD has laid on him the iniquity of us all. He was oppressed and afflicted, yet he did not open his mouth; he was led like a lamb to the slaughter, and as a sheep before its shearers is silent, so he did not open his mouth. By oppression and judgment he was taken away. Yet who of his generation protested? For he was cut off from the land of the living; for the transgression of my people he was punished. (Isaiah 53:5–8)

19. You did not choose me, but I chose you and appointed you so that you might go and bear fruit—fruit that will last—and so that whatever you ask in my name the Father will give you. This is my command: Love each other. (John 15:16–17)

20. Grace and peace to you from God our Father and the Lord Jesus Christ. Praise be to the God and Father of our Lord Jesus Christ, who has blessed us in the heavenly realms with every spiritual blessing in Christ. For he chose us in him before the creation of the world to be holy and blameless in his sight. In love he predestined us for adoption to sonship through Jesus Christ, in accordance with his pleasure and will—to the praise of his glorious grace, which he has freely given us in the One he loves. In him we have redemption through his blood, the forgiveness of sins, in accordance with the riches of God's grace that he lavished on us. With all wisdom and understanding, he made known to us the mystery of his will according to his good pleasure, which he purposed in Christ, to be put into effect when the times reach their fulfillment—to bring unity to all things in heaven and on earth under Christ. (Ephesians 1:2–10)

21. It was good for me to be afflicted so that I might learn your decrees. The law from your mouth is more precious to me than thousands of pieces of silver and gold. (Psalm 119:71–72)

"Though the mountains be shaken and the hills be removed, yet my unfailing love for you will not be shaken nor my covenant of peace be removed," says the LORD, who has compassion on you. "Afflicted city, lashed by storms and not comforted, I will rebuild you with stones of turquoise, your foundations with lapis lazuli. I will make your battlements of rubies, your gates of sparkling jewels, and all your walls of precious stones. All your children will be taught by the LORD, and great will be their peace." (Isaiah 54:10–13)

22. Then Peter came to Jesus and asked, "Lord, how many times shall I forgive my brother or sister who sins against me? Up to seven times?" Jesus answered, "I tell you, not seven times, but seventy-seven times." (Matthew 18:21–22)

You have heard that it was said, "Eye for eye, and tooth for tooth." But I tell you, do not resist an evil person. If anyone slaps you on the right cheek, turn to them the other cheek also. And if anyone wants to sue you and take your shirt, hand over your coat as well. If anyone forces you to go one mile, go with them two miles. Give to the one who asks you, and do not turn away from the one who wants to borrow from you. You have heard that it was said, "Love your neighbor and hate your enemy." But I tell you, love your enemies and pray for those who persecute you, that you may be children of your Father in heaven. He causes his sun to rise on the evil and the good, and sends rain on the righteous and the unrighteous. If you love those who love you, what reward will you get? Are not even the tax collectors doing that? And if you greet only your own people, what are you doing more than others? Do not even pagans do that? Be perfect, therefore, as your heavenly Father is perfect. (Matthew 5:38–48)

23. And when you pray, do not be like the hypocrites, for they love to pray standing in the synagogues and on the street corners to be seen by others. Truly I tell you, they have received their reward in full. But when you pray, go into your room, close the door and pray to your Father, who is unseen. Then your Father, who sees what is done in secret, will reward you. And when you pray, do not keep on babbling like pagans, for they think they will be heard because of their many words. Do not be like them, for your Father knows what you need before you ask him. This, then, is how you should pray: "Our Father in heaven, hallowed be your name, your kingdom come, your will be done, on earth as it is in heaven. Give us today our daily bread. And forgive us our debts, as we also have forgiven our debtors. And lead us not into temptation, but deliver us from the evil one." For if you forgive other people when they sin against you, your heavenly Father will also forgive you. But if you do not forgive others their sins, your Father will not forgive your sins. (Matthew 6:5–15)

24. Do good to your servant according to your word, LORD. Teach me knowledge and good judgment, for I trust your commands. Before I was afflicted I went astray, but now I obey your word. You are good, and what you do is good; teach me your decrees. Though the arrogant have smeared me with lies, I keep your precepts with all

my heart. Their hearts are callous and unfeeling, but I delight in your law. It was good for me to be afflicted so that I might learn your decrees. The law from your mouth is more precious to me than thousands of pieces of silver and gold. (Psalm 119:65–72)

25. In whom we have redemption, the forgiveness of sins. The Son is the image of the invisible God, the firstborn over all creation. For in him all things were created: things in heaven and on earth, visible and invisible, whether thrones or powers or rulers or authorities; all things have been created through him and for him. He is before all things, and in him all things hold together. And he is the head of the body, the church; he is the beginning and the firstborn from among the dead, so that in everything he might have the supremacy. For God was pleased to have all his fullness dwell in him, and through him to reconcile to himself all things, whether things on earth or things in heaven, by making peace through his blood, shed on the cross. Once you were alienated from God and were enemies in your minds because of your evil behavior. But now he has reconciled you by Christ's physical body through death to present you holy in his sight, without blemish and free from accusation. (Colossians 1:14–22)

26. Please see note 12.

But now apart from the law the righteousness of God has been made known, to which the Law and the Prophets testify. This righteousness is given through faith in Jesus Christ to all who believe. There is no difference between Jew and Gentile, for all have sinned and fall short of the glory of God, and all are justified freely by his grace through the redemption that came by Christ Jesus. God presented Christ as a sacrifice of atonement, through the shedding of his blood—to be received by faith. He did this to demonstrate his righteousness, because in his forbearance he had left the sins committed beforehand unpunished—he did it to demonstrate his righteousness at the present time, so as to be just and the one who justifies those who have faith in Jesus. Where, then, is boasting? It is excluded. Because of what law? The law that requires works? No, because of the law that requires faith. (Romans 3:21–27)

Now faith is confidence in what we hope for and assurance about what we do not see. (Hebrews 11:1)

And without faith it is impossible to please God, because anyone who comes to him must believe that he exists and that he rewards those who earnestly seek him. (Hebrews 11:6)

27. He then began to teach them that the Son of Man must suffer many things and be rejected by the elders, the chief priests and the teachers of the law, and that he must be killed and after three days rise again. He spoke plainly about this, and Peter took him aside and began to rebuke him. But when Jesus turned and looked at his disciples, he rebuked Peter. "Get behind me, Satan!" he said. "You do not have in mind the concerns of God, but merely human concerns." (Mark 8:31–33)

The seventy-two returned with joy and said, "Lord, even the demons submit to us in your name." He replied, "I saw Satan fall like lightning from heaven. I have given you authority to trample on snakes and scorpions and to overcome all the power of the enemy; nothing will harm you. However, do not rejoice that the spirits submit to you, but rejoice that your names are written in heaven." (Luke 10:17–20)

And giving joyful thanks to the Father, who has qualified you to share in the inheritance of his holy people in the kingdom of light. For he has rescued us from the dominion of darkness and brought us into the kingdom of the Son he loves. (Colossians 1:12–13)

28. For the Spirit God gave us does not make us timid, but gives us power, love and self-discipline. (2 Timothy 1:7)

29. Who has believed our message and to whom has the arm of the LORD been revealed? He grew up before him like a tender shoot, and like a root out of dry ground. He had no beauty or majesty to attract us to him, nothing in his appearance that we should desire him. He was despised and rejected by mankind, a man of suffering, and familiar with pain. Like one from whom people hide their faces he was despised, and we held him in low esteem. Surely he took up our pain and bore our suffering, yet we considered him punished by God, stricken by him, and afflicted. But he was pierced for our transgressions, he was crushed for our iniquities; the punishment that brought us peace was on him, and by his wounds we are healed. We all, like sheep, have gone astray, each of us has turned to our own way; and the LORD has laid on him the iniquity of us all. He was oppressed and afflicted, yet he did not open his mouth; he was led like a lamb to the slaughter, and as a sheep before its shearers is silent, so he did not open his mouth. By oppression and judgment he was taken away. Yet who of his generation protested? For he was cut off from the land of the living; for

the transgression of my people he was punished. He was assigned a grave with the wicked, and with the rich in his death, though he had done no violence, nor was any deceit in his mouth. Yet it was the LORD's will to crush him and cause him to suffer, and though the LORD makes his life an offering for sin, he will see his offspring and prolong his days, and the will of the LORD will prosper in his hand. After he has suffered, he will see the light of life and be satisfied; by his knowledge my righteous servant will justify many, and he will bear their iniquities. Therefore I will give him a portion among the great, and he will divide the spoils with the strong, because he poured out his life unto death, and was numbered with the transgressors. For he bore the sin of many, and made intercession for the transgressors. (Isaiah 53)

30. I am the true vine, and my Father is the gardener. He cuts off every branch in me that bears no fruit, while every branch that does bear fruit he prunes so that it will be even more fruitful. You are already clean because of the word I have spoken to you. Remain in me, as I also remain in you. No branch can bear fruit by itself; it must remain in the vine. Neither can you bear fruit unless you remain in me. I am the vine; you are the branches. If you remain in me and I in you, you will bear much fruit; apart from me you can do nothing. If you do not remain in me, you are like a branch that is thrown away and withers; such branches are picked up, thrown into the fire and burned. If you remain in me and my words remain in you, ask whatever you wish, and it will be done for you. This is to my Father's glory, that you bear much fruit, showing yourselves to be my disciples. As the Father has loved me, so have I loved you. Now remain in my love. If you keep my commands, you will remain in my love, just as I have

kept my Father's commands and remain in his love. I have told you this so that my joy may be in you and that your joy may be complete. My command is this: Love each other as I have loved you. Greater love has no one than this: to lay down one's life for one's friends. You are my friends if you do what I command. I no longer call you servants, because a servant does not know his master's business. Instead, I have called you friends, for everything that I learned from my Father I have made known to you. You did not choose me, but I chose you and appointed you so that you might go and bear fruit—fruit that will last—and so that whatever you ask in my name the Father will give you. This is my command: Love each other. If the world hates you, keep in mind that it hated me first. If you belonged to the world, it would love you as its own. As it is, you do not belong to the world, but I have chosen you out of the world. That is why the world hates you. Remember what I told you: A servant is not greater than his master. If they persecuted me, they will persecute you also. If they obeyed my teaching, they will obey yours also. They will treat you this way because of my name, for they do not know the one who sent me. If I had not come and spoken to them, they would not be guilty of sin; but now they have no excuse for their sin. Whoever hates me hates my Father as well. If I had not done among them the works no one else did, they would not be guilty of sin. As it is, they have seen, and yet they have hated both me and my Father. But this is to fulfill what is written in their Law: They hated me without reason. When the Advocate comes, whom I will send to you from the Father—the Spirit of truth who goes out from the Father—he will testify about me. And you also must testify, for you have been with me from the beginning. (John 15)

Though your contributions and donations Training Individuals Make Better Attitudes Inc

A section 501c3 not for profit organization, We can continue to educate, encourage and Inspire families in the community and all around the world. We train individuals in areas of stress and struggle. We believe if a family is trained in the areas In which they struggle, then that family can resolve their own issues.

If you want to support us please email us at: trainingindividuals2014@gmail.com

www.ingramcontent.com/pod-product-compliance
Lightning Source LLC
Chambersburg PA
CBHW020435290526
45785CB00002B/862